ABC of
Skin Cancer

ABC series

The revised and updated ABC series – written by specialists for non-specialists

- With over 40 titles, this extensive series provides a quick and dependable reference on a broad range of topics in all the major specialities

- An easy-to-use resource, covering the symptoms, investigations, treatment and management of conditions presenting in your day-to-day practice

- Full colour photographs and illustrations aid diagnosis and patient understanding of a condition

- Each book in the new series now offers links to further information and articles, and a new dedicated website provides even more support

- A highly illustrated, informative and practical source of knowledge for GPs, GP registrars, junior doctors, doctors in training and those in primary care

For further information on the entire ABC series, please visit:

www.abcbookseries.com

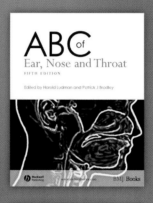

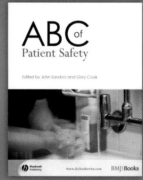

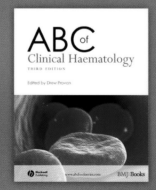

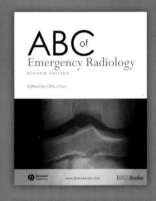

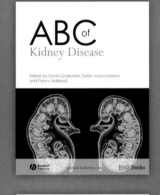

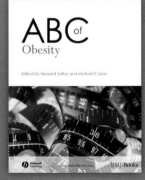

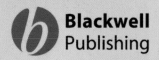

Blackwell Publishing

BMJ|Books

ABC of
Skin Cancer

EDITED BY

Sajjad Rajpar
Specialist Registrar in Dermatology
Skin Oncology Service, University Hospital Birmingham, Birmingham, UK

Jerry Marsden
Consultant Dermatologist
Skin Oncology Service, University Hospital Birmingham, Birmingham, UK

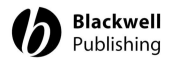
Blackwell
Publishing

BMJ|Books

Blackwell Publishing, Inc., 350 Main Street, Malden, Massachusetts 02148-5020, USA
Blackwell Publishing Ltd, 9600 Garsington Road, Oxford OX4 2DQ, UK
Blackwell Publishing Asia Pty Ltd, 550 Swanston Street, Carlton, Victoria 3053, Australia

1 2008

Library of Congress Cataloging-in-Publication Data

ABC of skin cancer / edited by Sajjad F. Rajpar, Jerry R. Marsden.
    p. ; cm.
  Includes bibliographical references and index.
  ISBN-13: 978-1-4051-6219-7 (alk. paper) 1. Skin--Cancer. I. Rajpar, Sajjad F. II. Marsden, Jerry R.
  [DNLM: 1. Skin Neoplasms. 2. Primary Health Care--methods. WR 500 A134 2008]

  RC280.S5A15 2008
  616.99'477--dc22

                        2007035840

ISBN: 978-1-4051-6219-7

A catalogue record for this title is available from the British Library

Cover image courtesy of Science Photo Library

Set in 9.25/12 pt Minion by Sparks, Oxford – www.sparkspublishing.com
Printed and bound by Printed and bound in Singapore by COS Printers Pte Ltd

Commissioning Editor: Mary Banks and Adam Gilbert
Editorial Assistant: Victoria Pittman and Laura McDonald
Production Controller: Rachel Edwards

For further information on Blackwell Publishing, visit our website:
www.blackwellpublishing.com

Contents

Contributors

Veronique Bataille
Senior Lecturer in Dermatology, The Royal London Hospital, London, UK

Graham Colver
Consultant Dermatologist, Chesterfield Royal Hospital NHS Foundation Trust, Chesterfield, UK

Karyn Fuller
Dermatology Resident Medical Officer, Women's and Children's Hospital, North Adelaide, Australia

F D Richard Hobbs
Professor of Primary Care and General Practice, The University of Birmingham, Edgbaston, Birmingham, UK

Marko Lens
Consultant Plastic and Reconstructive Surgeon, King's College, Genetic Epidemiology Unit, St Thomas' Hospital, London, UK

Jerry Marsden
Consultant Dermatologist, Skin Oncology Service, University Hospital Birmingham, Birmingham, UK

Richard Motley
Consultant in Dermatology and Cutaneous Surgery, University Hospital of Wales, Cardiff, UK

Julia A Newton-Bishop
Professor of Dermatology, Leeds Institute of Molecular Medicine, St James's University Hospital, Leeds, UK

Sajjad Rajpar
Specialist Registrar in Dermatology, Skin Oncology Service, University Hospital Birmingham, Birmingham, UK

Dev Shah
Specialist Registrar in Dermatology, University Hospital of Wales, Cardiff, UK

Lachlan Warren
Dermatologist, Women's and Children's Hospital, North Adelaide, Australia

Preface

The incidence of skin cancer in Europe, America and Australia has increased dramatically over the last few decades. Despite preventative public health measures, rates are projected to continue increasing. In the UK, skin cancers already account for one-quarter of all new malignancies, and 99% of these are basal cell carcinoma, squamous cell carcinoma and melanoma.

As a disease process, skin cancer lends itself well to prevention, early diagnosis and curative treatment; the leading environmental causative factor is known (ultraviolet radiation), phenotypic risk factors are well established and early diagnosis substantially improves the chance of cure. It is therefore surprising that education remains sparse on this group of cancers in both undergraduate and postgraduate medical curricula.

We have written this book to help fill this void. Our intention has been to provide a clinically orientated overview of the common skin cancers, focusing on clinical aspects of diagnosis and differential diagnosis, as well as practical management and preventative strategies relevant for the non-specialist. An insight into epidemiology, specialist management and rare skin cancers is also provided, as is a brief discussion of the genetic basis of skin cancers. The literature in this area is quite complex, but awareness of it is increasingly important in light of public and media interest in genetic testing.

This text is not intended to be an atlas of skin cancer, and the focus is not to encourage readers to 'match the lesion to the closest picture', which is tantamount to spot diagnosis. Given the huge spectrum of appearances of both benign and malignant lesions, this would neither be feasible (for example, tens of pictures would be required to depict the range in appearances of just seborrhoeic keratoses), nor a failsafe way of distinguishing benign from malignant lesions. Rather, we have tried to present concisely key diagnostic features and the variation in appearances of the most common lesions, focusing on the core clinical skills of history taking and examination to critically assess and triage lesions.

Although this text is in no way exhaustive, we hope it will be beneficial as an introductory guide. It should be useful as a continual source of reference for busy primary care practitioners who are faced with triaging patients with possible skin cancer, managing pre-cancerous lesions, educating on prevention, and supporting patients during and after skin cancer treatment. Trainees in dermatology, doctors from allied specialties, junior doctors, medical students and nurses may also find this text relevant.

Sajjad Rajpar, Jerry Marsden

CHAPTER 1

The epidemiology, aetiology and prevention of melanoma

Julia A Newton-Bishop

OVERVIEW

- Over the last three decades, incidence rates of melanoma in the UK have increased every year. Increments in mortality have been smaller, and melanoma accounts for 1–2% of total cancer deaths.

- Incidence of melanoma is greater in females, whereas mortality from melanoma is greater in males.

- Melanoma is a cancer seen predominantly in pale-skinned people and the dominant behavioural risk factor in Europe is acute intermittent sun exposure on sunny holidays.

- Risk factors for melanoma include red hair and freckles, skin which burns in the sun and a positive family history.

- The Atypical Mole syndrome is a phenotype associated with the presence of over 100 moles and two or more atypical moles. This is the most potent phenotypic risk factor for melanoma.

- Rare families exist in which multiple cases of melanoma occur and a proportion of these families have hereditary mutations in the *CDKN2A* gene.

- Behaviours that protect against strong sunlight should be encouraged among patients at risk of melanoma. A simple message is: 'don't burn, don't tan'.

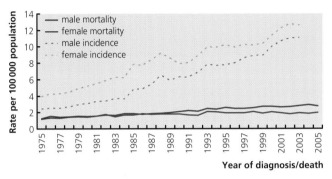

Fig. 1.1 Age-standardized (European) incidence and mortality rates of melanoma by sex in Great Britain between 1975 and 2005.

Melanoma is the eighth most common malignancy in the UK. In 2003, there were 8114 new cases and 1777 deaths. Incidence rates have increased every year for the last three decades, faster than that of any other major cancer, making melanoma an increasing public health concern. Despite this, increments in mortality have been smaller, and melanoma accounts for only 1–2% of total cancer deaths in the UK. One-third of patients are under the age of 50, and approximately 15 years of life are lost for each death, placing melanoma amongst the top five cancer causes of lost life-years.

Epidemiology

In the UK, the incidence of melanoma has more than tripled over the last 25 years to age-standardized rates of 11.1 per 100 000 in men and 12.6 per 100 000 in women in 2003 (Figure 1.1). The increase in incidence has been greatest for melanoma under 1 mm in Breslow thickness. It has been proposed that this increasing trend may be an epiphenomenon attributed to earlier detection, better surveillance and changes in diagnostic criteria. However, available evidence suggests much of the rising incidence is real.

Mortality rates have also significantly risen over the last 25 years (Fig. 1.1), but at a much slower pace as tumours < 1 mm in Breslow thickness have a good prognosis. In contrast to incidence, mortality is greater in men, with male deaths outnumbering female deaths almost twofold. The rise in melanoma mortality has been greatest among men aged >65 years, who present late with thick (> 4 mm in Breslow depth) advanced tumours that have a poor prognosis. Reasons for this include the tendency for melanoma to be located on the back in males where they are hard to see, lack of self-examination and a tendency for not reporting changing moles.

Risk factors

The most common types of primary cutaneous melanoma – superficial spreading melanoma (Fig. 9.3), nodular melanoma (Fig. 9.4) and lentigo maligna melanoma (Fig. 9.5) – are cancers of white-skinned people and are associated with a number of well-established risk factors (Table 1.1). Rarely, melanoma occurs on the palms and soles, nail apparatus and genital and sinonasal mucosa (Fig. 9.6). These rare subtypes are equally common in all ethnic groups irrespective of skin colour, and are of unknown aetiology.

Certain heritable traits such as red hair and freckles are associated with an increased relative risk for melanoma of about 3. The most potent risk factor, however, is the presence of increased numbers of moles (benign melanocytic naevi) and the presence of bigger moles with an irregular or ill-defined edge, known as atypical moles. Moles are acquired proliferative lesions, which appear from early childhood until mid-adult life, when they start to reduce in number. In-

Table 1.1 Risk factors for melanoma. Note that many of these factors are interdependent and have not been subject to multivariate analysis, so cannot be used to compute the precise risk of melanoma for a given individual.

Risk factor	Relative risk
Physical characteristics	
Fair skin (that burns easily and does not tan)	1.4
Light eye colour	1.6
Red or light-coloured hair	1.4–3.5
Freckles	1.9–3.5
Number of benign melanocytic naevi (>2 mm)	
11–50	1.7–1.9
51–100	3.2–3.7
>100	7.6–11
Number of atypical moles	
1–4	1.6–7.3
>5	5.7–8.6
Family history	
Melanoma in one first-degree relative	2.4–3.0
Melanoma in three or more first-degree relatives	35–70
Others	
Single blistering sunburn	2.0–3.0
Regular sunbed use (starting under the age of 35)	1.8
Higher social class	3.0

dividuals living in hot countries, such as Australia, have more moles then those living in Europe, implying that they are induced by sun exposure. However, twin studies provide good evidence that the number of moles is also determined genetically. As large numbers

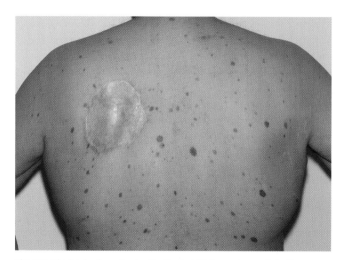

Fig. 1.2 The back of a patient with Atypical Mole syndrome. Note the scar from wider excision of a melanoma.

Box 1.1 Atypical Mole syndrome

One definition of the Atypical Mole syndrome is the presence of two or more of the features listed here. Using this definition, 2% of the UK population have the Atypical Mole syndrome and are at a greater risk of developing melanoma.

- ≥100 naevi >2 mm (≥50 if aged <20 years or >50 years)
- 2 or more atypical naevi
- 1 or more naevi on the buttocks
- 2 or more naevi on the dorsal feet

---

of moles are a risk factor for melanoma, it is hypothesized that that mole genes are also low-risk melanoma susceptibility genes. Two per cent of the UK population have the Atypical Mole syndrome (Fig. 1.2, Box 1.1), which is a phenotype associated with both large numbers of moles (more than 100 moles >2 mm in diameter) and moles which are atypical (being larger than 5 mm in diameter with an irregular shape and colour). Patients with the Atypical Mole syndrome have a significantly increased risk of melanoma.

Sun exposure

Ultraviolet (UV) B accounts for 5% of the UV radiation in natural sunlight and is the major cause of skin cancer and sunburn. UVA accounts for 95% and is contributory. Melanoma is most common in people who are pale skinned and who tend to burn in the sun. This is evidence for sun exposure as its environmental cause. The incidence of melanoma is highest where fair-skinned people live at low latitudes such as Australia, which is further evidence for sun exposure as causal. The recent increase in incidence has been attributed to changes in social attitude and behaviour over the last century. Past social convention prevented exposure of much of the skin. This has now changed, with large proportions of the population exposing nearly all of their skin intermittently to sudden large doses of sunlight (Fig. 1.3). Epidemiological studies have supported the view that the key behavioural factor for melanoma is acute intermittent exposure to strong sunlight, such as on sunny holidays. Case–control data have also repeatedly identified sunburn as a risk factor for melanoma, especially in early life. Chronic low-dose over-exposure seen in outdoor workers does not appear to be so clearly related to melanoma risk in Europe, but may still be causal in a proportion of cases. This sort of over exposure is more closely related to the risk of cutaneous squamous cell carcinoma (SCC).

Sunbeds

There is strong evidence to suggest that exposure to sunbeds increases the risk of melanoma and SCC. A recent systematic review concluded the relative risk for melanoma was 1.8 among regular

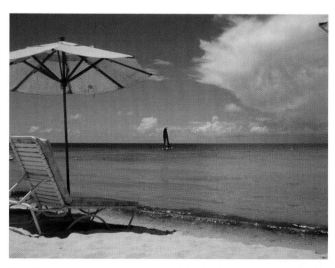

Fig. 1.3 The type of sun exposure which is held to be most likely to produce melanoma in Europe is short, intense exposure in fair-skinned indoor workers, of the type seen on sunny holidays, rather than chronic cumulative sun exposure.

users of sunbeds who start before the age of 35. This is concerning, as up to 7% of the UK population may use sunbeds. Proponents of the cosmetic tanning industry continue to argue that sunbed use is required to maintain adequate vitamin D levels and an indoor tan protects against sunburn from subsequent exposure to sunlight. Although winter vitamin D levels may be inadequate in some individuals, alternative sources of vitamin D are more appropriate. Furthermore, skin that has been tanned using sunbeds (which emit a greater UVA to UVB ratio than natural sunlight) is less protected from sunburn than an equivalent natural tan.

Family history and melanoma susceptibility genes

A positive family history of melanoma is also a risk factor for melanoma. A study from the Swedish Cancer Registry estimated the standardized incidence ratio (approximating to relative risk) for melanoma to be 2.4 for offspring if one parent had a melanoma and 3.0 for a sibling. Rare families exist in which large numbers of cases of melanoma occur, and the majority of these families have hereditary mutations in a gene called *CDKN2A*, which codes for two proteins, P16 and P14ARF. Even rarer families have mutations in a gene coding for *CDK4*. Other high-risk genes remain to be identified.

In most *CDKN2A* mutation-positive families in the UK and Australia, family members appear to be at increased risk of melanoma alone. In families with *CDKN2A* mutations living in North America and in some parts of Europe, there is also an increased risk of pancreatic cancer (Fig. 1.4). The frequency of CDKN2A mutations is 20–40% in families where there are three or more affected first-degree relatives, and < 5% if there are only two. This means that hereditary mutations are responsible for a very small proportion of melanoma. The penetrance of CDKN2A mutations, and factors which moderate the penetrance, are poorly understood. Gene testing for mutations is therefore of limited clinical utility at present and is best restricted to the research setting.

Racial variation

Although melanoma occurs most commonly in individuals with white skin, it can occur in all races. Recent American data have shown the age-adjusted incidence of melanoma per 100 000 in different ethnic subtypes to be 18.9 in Whites, 4.0 in Hispanics, 1.5 in Far East Asians and 1.0 in Blacks. The lower incidence of melanoma in ethnic groups is attributed to the protective effects of epidermal melanin against UV radiation, which, in very dark black skin, affords a Sun Protection Factor (SPF) equivalent to 13.4. The majority of melanoma in non-White populations occurs on sun-protected sites such as the palms, soles and mucosal surfaces. However, some data have shown that lighter-skinned Hispanics tend to develop melanoma on sun-exposed sites in a similar distribution to Whites compared with dark-skinned Hispanics. This suggests that the degree of pigmentation in ethnic groups may influence the site and incidence of melanoma. This is of particular relevance given the increasing proportion of mixed races who have intermediate pigmentation in Western countries.

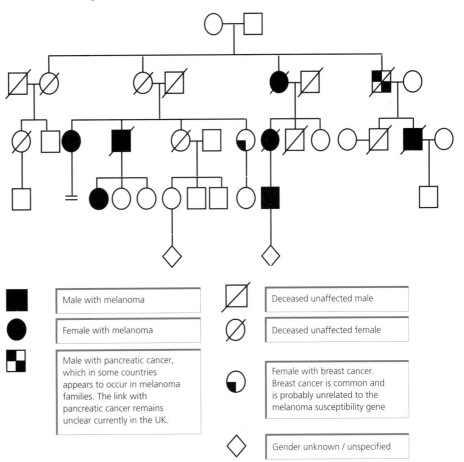

■	Male with melanoma
●	Female with melanoma
(quartered square)	Male with pancreatic cancer, which in some countries appears to occur in melanoma families. The link with pancreatic cancer remains unclear currently in the UK.
⊘ (square)	Deceased unaffected male
⊘ (circle)	Deceased unaffected female
(circle, part-filled)	Female with breast cancer. Breast cancer is common and is probably unrelated to the melanoma susceptibility gene
◇	Gender unknown / unspecified

Fig. 1.4 This family tree illustrates the pattern of cancer seen in families with hereditary mutations in the *CDKN2A* gene, which are transmitted in a dominant fashion with incomplete penetrance.

Primary prevention

It is likely that the incidence of melanoma can be reduced by widespread reduction in exposure to strong sunlight, particularly by children and young adults. Complete sun avoidance is clearly impractical – a simple message to patients is 'don't burn, don't tan'. This can be achieved by following the SunSmart Code (Box 1.2). When a sunscreen is used, a broad-spectrum product that protects against UVA and UVB, with an SPF rating of ≥ 30 should be chosen.

Sunscreens

Case-controlled studies into sunscreens have not consistently supported their beneficial effects in reducing melanoma. This is probably because many of these studies are subjected to significant confounding and bias, and were conducted before newer, more efficacious and better accepted sunscreens were introduced. The SPF rating of a sunscreen is the factor by which it protects from UVB erythema (early sunburn) and is based on controlled phototesting of untanned skin at an even application thickness of $2\,\text{mg/cm}^2$. For example, a product with an SPF of 15 allows an untanned individual to withstand 15 times the amount of UVB before developing erythema. In reality, most individuals do not use enough sunscreen, typically applying only $0.5–1.0\,\text{mg/cm}^2$. Application thickness is often uneven, may decrease after water exposure, and re-application may be inadequate. Consequently, the effective SPF of a sunscreen may be one-third of the nominal SPF. When sunscreens were first popularized in the early 1980s, the median SPF was 4–6. Some older sunscreens permitted high levels of UVA exposure to facilitate tanning and avoid burning, which might paradoxically have increased risk of skin cancer. Current sunscreens are more effective, protecting against UVA as well as UVB with typical SPF values of ≥ 20. The impact of these newer sunscreens on melanoma prevention may take several decades to be demonstrated.

Sun-protective clothing

The degree to which clothing impedes penetration of UVR is known as the Ultraviolet Protection Factor (UPF) and is based on the fibre content and weave, colour, finishing process and the presence of additives. Almost 90% of summer clothing has a UPF of > 10, and 80% has a UPF of > 15. Clothing is therefore a reliable and effective method of photoprotection, and should be encouraged.

Box 1.2 **The SunSmart Code – from SunSmart, the UK's national skin cancer prevention campaign (http://info. cancerresearchuk.org/healthyliving/sunsmart). The authors and editors would advise that if a sunscreen is used, it should block ultraviolet (UV) A and UVB with a Sun Protection Factor of ≥30.**

Spend time in the shade between 11 and 3
Make sure you never burn
Aim to cover up with a t-shirt, hat and sunglasses
Remember to take extra care with children
Then use factor 15+ sunscreen

Also, report mole changes or unusual skin growths promptly to your doctor.

Further reading

Bishop JA, Wachsmuth RC, Harland M *et al.* Genotype/phenotype and penetrance studies in melanoma families with germline CDK2NA mutations. J Invest Dermatol 2000; 114:28–33.

Cancer Research UK. UK Malignant Melanoma statistics. Available at http://info.cancerresearchuk.org/cancerstats/types/melanoma/?a=5441

Diffey BL. Is daily use of sunscreens of benefit in the U.K.? Br J Dermatol 2002; 146:659–62.

Downing A, Newton-Bishop JA, Forman D. Recent trends in cutaneous malignant melanoma in the Yorkshire region of England; incidence, mortality and survival in relation to stage of disease, 1993–2003. Br J Cancer 2006; 95:91–5.

Gandini S, Sera F, Cattaruzza MS, Pasquini P, Picconi O, Boyle P *et al.* Meta-analysis of risk factors for cutaneous melanoma: II. Sun exposure. Eur J Cancer 2005; 41:45–60.

Gloster HM, Neal K. Skin cancer in skin of color. J Am Acad Dermatol 2006; 55:741–60.

Hemminki K, Zhang H, Czene K. Familial and attributable risks in cutaneous melanoma: effects of proband and age. J Invest Dermatol 2003; 120:217–23.

International Agency for Research on Cancer Working Group on artificial ultraviolet (UV) light and skin cancer. The association of use of sunbeds with cutaneous malignant melanoma and other skin cancers: a systematic review. Int J Cancer 2007; 120:1116–22.

Newton-Bishop A, Harland M, Randerson-Moor J, Bishop DT. The management of familial melanoma. Lancet Oncology 2006; in press.

CHAPTER 2

The epidemiology, aetiology and prevention of non-melanoma skin cancer

Veronique Bataille, Marko Lens, Sajjad Rajpar

OVERVIEW

- Non-melanoma skin cancer (NMSC) is a collective term for basal cell carcinoma (BCC) and squamous cell carcinoma (SCC).

- NMSCs are the commonest cancers to affect White populations, and incidence in the UK is increasing at 3–8% per year.

- Individuals who are fair skinned, have light eye colour and a tendency to sunburn are at the highest risk of developing NMSC.

- Exposure to ultraviolet (UV) radiation is the most important causative factor in NMSC. Episodic high-intensity UV exposure in early life is important for the development of BCC, whereas SCC is most closely associated with the total amount of lifetime UV exposure.

- The genetic basis of NMSC is not yet fully understood, but many genes are likely to be involved.

- Actinic keratoses have very low risk of progression to SCC.

- Photoprotective measures have been shown to reduce the incidence of SCC, but not of BCC.

Non-melanoma skin cancer (NMSC) is a collective term for basal cell carcinoma (BCC) and squamous cell carcinoma (SCC). They are the commonest epidermal malignancies and the most common types of cancer in the UK with a reported 67 500 episodes in 2003. Many other types of non-melanoma cutaneous malignancies are recognized (Table 2.1), though these are rare and not dealt with further in this chapter (see Chapter 14). The registration of NMSC varies widely across cancer registries, and several tumours, particularly those that are treated without histological sampling (such as superficial BCC), remain unreported. The true incidence of NMSC in the UK is therefore much higher, estimated to be 100 000 per year and increasing at an annual rate of 3–8%. Although the incidence is high, NMSC accounts for < 400 deaths a year – the majority related to metastatic SCC. The importance of NMSC is often disregarded due to the relatively good prognosis, although delayed diagnosis and suboptimal management can lead to disfigurement and loss of life. The large number of cases and the trends for increasing incidence underline the morbidity and economic burden of this growing public health problem.

Basal cell carcinoma

BCC is the most common form of skin cancer in White individuals in temperate climates, accounting for 80% of NMSC. BCCs are slow growing and invade local tissues; metastasis is extremely rare. The clinical features of BCCs are discussed in Chapter 6.

Epidemiology

The registration of BCC is poor in many countries despite its high incidence. One reason is that BCCs may be treated by different clinical specialists with methods, such as cryotherapy, that may preclude histological confirmation. These limitations are reflected in the reported annual incidence rates in Europe, which range from 50 to 130 per 100 000 (Table 2.2). The annual incidence in Australia is much higher, ranging from 800 to 1500 per 100 000. The difference in incidence provides evidence for the causative role of ultraviolet (UV) radiation. The mean age at diagnosis is 60 years, although over the

Table 2.1 Types of primary skin cancer and their cell of origin.

Cancer	Cell of origin
Basal cell carcinoma	Uncertain: basal cell keratinocyte or follicular stem cells
Squamous cell carcinoma	Keratinocyte
Melanoma	Melanocyte
Cutaneous lymphoma	Lymphocyte
Merkel cell carcinoma	Neuroendocrine cell
Appendageal tumours	Cells in the hair follicle, sebaceous glands and sweat glands
Angiosarcoma	Endothelial cell
Sarcoma, DFSP	Fibroblast, smooth muscle myocite

Typically, non-melanoma skin cancer refers to basal cell carcinoma and squamous cell carcinoma, though there are several uncommon types of skin cancer besides melanoma. DFSP: dermatofibrosarcoma protuberans.

Table 2.2 Reported age-standardized incidence rates (world standard population, per 100 000 person-years) in selected Western European registries.

Registry	Year	Age-standardized incidence rates (per 100 000)	
		Male	Female
Finland	1991–1995	49	45
Hull, UK	1991	116	104
Vaud, Switzerland	1991–1992	69	62
Wales, UK	1998	128	105
Schleswig-Holstein, Germany	1998–2001	54	44
Eindhoven, the Netherlands	1998–2000	63	58

Box 2.1 **Risk factors for basal cell carcinoma**

- Patient factors
  a. Fair skin
  b. Light eye colour
  c. Red or blond hair
  d. Family history of BCC
  e. Multiple atypical naevi
  f. Immunosuppression

- Environmental factors
  a. Low latitude
  b. Episodic high-intensity sun exposure
  c. Previous radiotherapy
  d. Exposure to arsenic

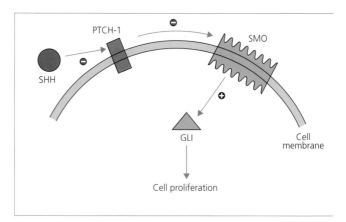

Fig. 2.1 Molecular pathogenesis of basal cell carcinoma (BCC). The PTCH-sonic hedgehog signalling network is up-regulated by loss of function mutations in PTCH-1 (patched homologue 1), and gain for function mutations in SHH (sonic hedgehog), SMO (smoothened protein) and the GLI transcription factors. +, Stimulatory effect; –, inhibitory effect.

last 10 years there has been a notable increase in BCC among younger individuals, especially females in the 20–40-year age group.

Risk factors

As with other skin cancers, exposure to UV radiation is the most important risk factor for developing BCC (Box 2.1). BCC mainly affects individuals who have a tendency to sunburn, such as those with fair skin and light eye colour. The exact relationship between sun exposure and the development of BCC is unclear, and certainly more complex than for SCC. For example, relatively sun-protected areas such as behind the ear are affected disproportionately more than heavily sun-exposed areas such as the helix of the ear. In addition, patients who develop BCC tend to have less photodamage (including actinic keratoses, solar lentigines and photoageing) compared with patients who develop SCC. These observations suggest that intermittent sun exposure in childhood and early adulthood is more relevant, as for melanoma, than cumulative UV exposure as with SCC. Less common risk factors include exposure to radiation, arsenic and immunosuppression. Identical twin pairs have been reported to develop BCC at a similar age and at similar sites, suggesting genetic susceptibility plays a strong role. Other epigenetic factors which are yet to be determined are also likely to play a role.

Genetics

The discovery in 1994 of the *PTCH* gene on chromosome 9q was a major genetic breakthrough in the molecular pathogenesis of BCC. Germ-line mutations in this gene lead to an autosomal dominant transmission of the Gorlin syndrome, which is characterized by multiple BCCs from an early age, broad nasal bridge with hypertelorism, jaw cysts, palmar pits and bifid ribs. Somatic mutations that amplify the PTCH-sonic hedgehog signalling network (Fig. 2.1), a major cell cycle regulatory pathway, have since been discovered to be important events in sporadic BCC. Other polymorphisms may also play a role, including the melanocortin-1 receptor (*MC1R*) gene, glutathione methyl transferase (*GSTT*) gene and DNA repair genes.

Squamous cell carcinoma

SCC is the second most common form of skin cancer, accounting in the UK for about 20% of all NMSC. The clinical features of SCC are discussed in Chapter 5.

Epidemiology

SCC incidence demonstrates geographical variation, increasing strikingly at lower latitudes. Incidence is as high as 1000 per 100 000 person-years in White residents of tropical Australia, compared with 30.2 in males and 14.1 in females per 100 000 person-years in Sweden. The incidence of SCC also appears to increase exponentially after the age of 60 years, affecting twice as many men as women. In contrast to BCC, SCC tends to be more aggressive, as it is not only locally invasive but can also metastasize to lymph nodes and more distant organs. Annual mortality rates from SCC were 0.29 per 100 000 in Rhode Island between 1988 and 2000.

Risk factors

Cumulative lifetime exposure to UV radiation in fair-skinned individuals is the most important risk factor for the development of SCC (Box 2.2). Solar-induced SCC typically develops on an exposed site such as the head, neck and backs of the hands either *de novo* or from precursor lesions such as actinic keratosis (AK) and Bowen's disease. Although SCCs are much more likely to occur in patients with large numbers of AKs, the rate of transformation to SCC of individual AK lesions is very low.

Chronically immunosuppressed patients are between 65 to 250 times more susceptible to developing SCC; this is likely to be related to human papillomavirus infection. Other predisposing factors for SCC include exposure to ionizing radiation and chemical carcinogens such as betel nuts (particularly for SCC of the mouth and lips). SCC can also arise in areas of chronic scarring due to burns (known as Marjolin's ulcer) and in areas that are chronically affected by certain inflammatory skin disorders such as lichen sclerosus, ulcers and sinus tracts.

Genetics

The exact genetic steps involved in transforming normal skin to SCC, either directly or via intermediate clinical lesions such as AKs, are not clear. The accumulation of several genetic alterations and instabilities, resulting from direct UV damage to DNA, is believed to create highly complex karyotypes with many aberrations. So far, no single gene has been shown to be consistently altered in SCC, al-

Box 2.2 Risk factors for SCC

- Patient factors
  a. Fair skin
  b. Light eye colour
  c. Red or blond hair
  d. Male gender
  e. Presence of many actinic keratoses and Bowen's disease lesions
  f. Previous non-melanoma skin cancer
  g. Immunosuppression
  h. Burn scars, chronic ulcers, sinuses
  i. Chronic cutaneous inflammation, e.g. lichen sclerosus, erosive lichen planus
  j. Uncircumcised male (penile SCC)
  k. Genetic disorders, e.g. oculocutaneous albinism

- Environmental factors
  a. Exposure to ultraviolet light including natural sunlight, sunbeds and phototherapy
  b. Previous radiotherapy
  c. Exposure to arsenic and polycyclic aromatic hydrocarbons

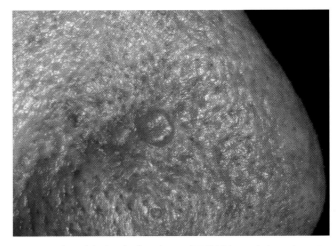

Fig. 2.2 Early nodular basal cell carcinoma (BCC). This papule is pearlescent, has surface telangiectasias and measures only 2.5 mm in diameter. Detecting BCC at an early stage reduces morbidity.

though aberrations in the p53, RAS Retinoblastoma and CDKNA2/p16^{INK4a} pathways are frequently reported.

Racial variation in NMSC

Skin cancers are significantly less common in Black and Asian individuals; one study has estimated them to occur 70 times less frequently. SCC is the most common skin cancer in these ethnic groups, accounting for two-thirds of cases. Most lesions are unrelated to UV radiation, occurring on sun-protected sites such as the lower limbs, anogenital area and hair-bearing scalp. BCCs are less common, but predominantly affect older individuals on the sun-exposed sites of the head and neck. This would suggest that exposure to intense and prolonged UV radiation has a significant role to play in the small number of BCCs that occur in pigmented skin types.

Prevention of NMSC

Both BCC and SCC are associated with excessive exposure to UV radiation, both natural (from sunlight) and artificial (from sunbeds). BCC is associated with episodic intense exposure in childhood and young adulthood, whereas SCC correlates better with cumulative sun exposure. Hence, suitable measures at limiting exposure to these patterns of

UV radiation should logically reduce levels of NMSC. Results from a recent Australian randomized controlled trial have demonstrated that risk of SCC is reduced by regular sunscreen use, and this protective effect is apparent up to 8 years after cessation of the intervention. There was no reduction in BCC incidence. Several other preventative strategies have been investigated, including supplementation with selenium, carotenoids and vitamin E and reduced-fat diets. However, none has shown consistent benefit. Early diagnosis (Fig. 2.2) and prompt intervention continue to be an important aspect of minimizing morbidity from NMSC. Education programmes should therefore include messages to the public on recognizing and reporting new, fixed and abnormal skin growths.

Further reading

Boukamp P. Non-melanoma skin cancer: what drives tumor development and progression? Carcinogenesis 2005; 26:4657–67.

de Vries E, Marieke L, Maarten B *et al*. Rapid and continuous increases in incidence rates of basal cell carcinoma in the Southeast Netherlands since 1973. J Invest Dermatol 2004; 123:634–8.

Hemminki K, Zhang H, Czene K. Time trends and familial risks in squamous cell carcinoma of the skin. Arch Dermatol 2003;139:885–9.

Lear W, Dahlke E, Murray CA. Basal cell carcinoma: review of epidemiology, pathogenesis, and associated risk factors. J Cutan Med Surg 2007; 11:19–30.

van der Pols JC, Williams GM, Pandeya N *et al*. Prolonged prevention of squamous cell carcinoma of the skin by regular sunscreen use. Cancer Epidemiol Biomarkers Prev 2006;15:2546–8.

CHAPTER 3

The role of the primary care team in the management of skin cancer

F D Richard Hobbs

OVERVIEW

- The primary care team has a pivotal role in the early diagnosis of skin cancer. This has the greatest impact on prognosis.

- Other roles of the primary care team include educating the public on ways to reduce risk of skin cancer, promoting skin self-examination in individuals at high risk of skin cancer, and follow-up of skin cancer patients.

- In the UK, the National Institute of Health and Clinical Excellence (NICE) guidance on skin cancer emphasizes that most pre-cancerous skin lesions (such as actinic keratosis and Bowen's disease) and some low-risk basal cell carcinomas (BCC) may be treated in the community. Undiagnosed lesions, lesions suspicious of malignancy, squamous cell carcinoma, high-risk BCC and melanoma should be referred to a specialist. Practices should have access to dedicated, rapid-access skin cancer clinics to facilitate this.

As with most cancers, the key role for primary care is early diagnosis and referral, or appropriate immediate management, of suspicious presenting lesions (Fig. 3.1). Perhaps of equivalent importance, particularly in countries with high incidence rates, is the role of primary care in educating the public on ways to reduce risk of skin cancer, and on how to effectively self-examine. The primary care team may also be involved in the follow-up of skin cancer patients. The role of primary care, and its integration with secondary care, has been clearly defined in the UK by the National Institute of Health and Clinical Excellence (NICE).

Diagnosing skin cancer

The most important determinant of outcome of many types of cancer remains the point at which the diagnosis is confirmed – the earlier the diagnosis and subsequent curative treatment the more likely it is that the prognosis will be improved. Since most skin lesions will present initially in the community, primary care has a pivotal role in early and accurate diagnosis.

Non-melanoma skin cancer

Non-melanoma skin cancer (NMSC) presents most commonly in those > 50 years old. However, in high-incidence areas such as Australia, NMSC occurs at an earlier age and disease in the 30s is not unusual. Increased age at presentation may therefore increase the

likelihood that a skin lesion could be cancerous (Box 3.1). However, the age range at presentation is wide. Site of lesions may similarly increase likelihood of cancer, but again cannot be used to exclude malignancy. Indeed, there are differences in reported rates for sites of cancer when series based on hospital-treated are compared with general practice-treated populations. For example, whereas around 75% of basal cell carcinomas (BCC) are located on the head and neck in hospital series, this is the site in around 40% of cases treated in Australian general practice, where higher rates of BCC are reported on the shoulder and trunk. The explanation is likely to be that trunk BCCs tend to be of the superficial subtype, not near important anatomy and easier to treat. The overall implications for general practice are that skin lesions that present with suspicious features should be referred for diagnosis regardless of age and site of the lesion.

Melanoma

For pigmented lesions, there is greater urgency over the time to diagnosis and importance of complete excision for diagnosis (Box 3.2). In the UK, practices can urgently refer to dedicated rapid-access skin cancer clinics for specialist assessment. NICE guidance specifically requires lesions suspicious of melanoma to be referred and not managed in primary care. This is because accurate diagnosis requires careful integration of the history and clinical findings and specialist histopathology of a completely excised lesion.

Managing skin cancer

In the UK, any doctor who treats skin cancer is required to comply with the NICE guidance on skin cancer, which brings skin cancer care into line with other areas of the NHS Cancer Plan (Box 3.3). The emphasis is for most pre-cancerous skin lesions and some low-risk BCCs to be treated in the community, and for melanoma, squamous cell carcinoma (SCC), high-risk BCC, undiagnosed lesions and lesions suspicious of malignancy to be referred to a specialist.

Preventing skin cancer

Sun avoidance is especially important during childhood and teenage years, since a high proportion of lifetime risk results from ultraviolet radiation exposure during this period. Simple sun avoidance advice (Box 1.2) should be provided opportunistically to patients at risk of skin cancer (Box 3.4), particularly to individuals who are

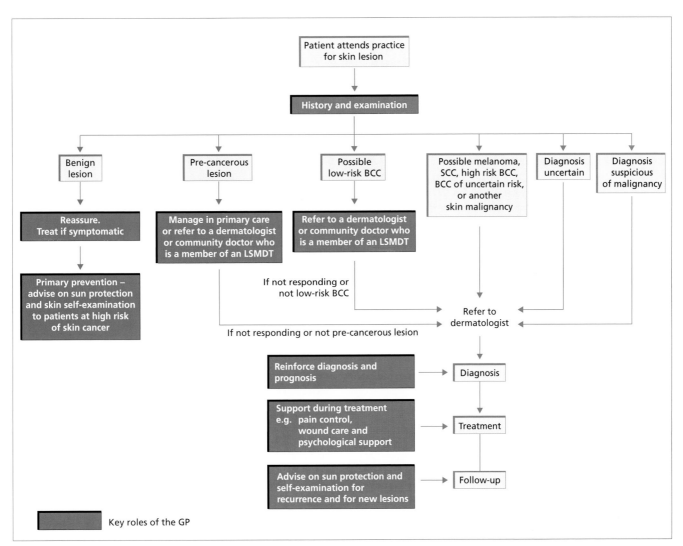

Fig. 3.1 Flow chart showing the key roles for the UK general practitioner (green) in diagnosing, managing and preventing skin cancer. LSMDT: Local skin cancer multidisciplinary team.

Box 3.1 Lesions that are most commonly confused with non-melanoma skin cancer

- Pre-cancerous lesions, e.g. actinic keratosis and Bowen's disease
- Seborrhoeic keratosis
- Intradermal naevus
- Cyst
- Sebaceous hyperplasia
- Dermatofibroma

Box 3.2 Lesions that are most commonly confused with melanoma

- Seborrhoeic keratosis
- Junctional, compound and intradermal naevi
- Atypical mole
- Simple lentigo
- Dermatofibroma

---

fair skinned or burn easily and in low- or high-altitude environments.

Public education

Public education programmes on the risks of skin cancer should involve the media, and specific advice given to children and teenagers. General public education programmes in the UK have been associated with reductions in melanoma thickness and therefore improved prognosis. However, it is unclear if this relationship is causal, as similar trends are present in areas without education campaigns, and there is concern that the increased volume of referrals to specialists may have displaced other specialist services. Primary care can play an important role in terms of opportunistic advice to patients attending routine clinics. This should comprise information available in waiting rooms and specific (and repeated) preventive advice offered opportunistically during routine consultations, particularly to parents about their children.

Primary care has been involved in skin cancer prevention programmes in Australia since the early 1960s. Observational data suggest

---

Box 3.3 Key recommendations from the UK NICE guidance on skin cancer

- Two levels of multidisciplinary teams should be established by cancer networks: LSMDTs (local hospital skin cancer multidisciplinary teams) and SSMDTs (specialist skin cancer multidisciplinary teams).
- All health professionals who treat patients with any type of skin cancer should be members of one of these teams, whether they work in the community or in the hospital setting.
- People with pre-cancerous skin lesions should be either treated entirely by their GP or referred for diagnosis, treatment and follow-up to doctors working in the community who are members of the LSMDT.
- Patients with low-risk basal cell carcinomas (BCCs) should be diagnosed, treated and followed up by doctors working in the community as part of the LSMDT or a dermatologist.
- Doctors working in the community who are members of the LSMDT are typically general practitioners (GPs) with a specialist interest in Dermatology, though in the future this may include community dermatologists.
- All patients with a suspicious pigmented skin lesion, with a skin lesion that may be a high-risk BCC, a squamous cell carcinoma or a melanoma, or where the diagnosis is uncertain, should be referred to a dermatologist.

Box 3.4 Simple factors can be used to increase public awareness of identifying individuals at higher risk of melanoma, reducing risk from melanoma and recognizing early signs of melanoma

- Identifying individuals at higher risk of melanoma
  - Fair skin
  - Red hair
  - Tendency to freckles
  - Multiple moles (>20)
  - Large moles with irregular edge or colour (atypical moles)
  - History of sunburn
  - Family history of melanoma
- Reducing risk from melanoma
  - Sun avoidance behaviour
  - Avoidance of artificial ultraviolet light, e.g. sunbeds
- Recognizing early signs of melanoma. Check skin regularly for:
  - Change in shape of mole
  - Change in size of mole
  - Change in colour of mole
  - New lesion that looks odd

that these programmes have contributed to a reduction in skin cancer rates in Australians under the age of 60 years. Outside Australia, preliminary data show that nurse-led and media-led patient education programmes improve rates of skin self-examination, reduce fears of skin cancer and improve knowledge and sun avoidance. More data on the utility of such interventions in the generality of practice settings are needed.

Screening for melanoma

The much higher incidence of melanoma in Australia has led to educational strategies to increase public awareness of risk, primary prevention measures to reduce risk, earlier recognition of abnormal signs in skin lesions, and thus earlier diagnosis (Box 3.4).

The relative rarity of melanoma outside Australia means that population screening is not cost-effective. However, preliminary studies suggest that selective screening by using practitioner- or patient-administered skin cancer risk scores can identify a cohort of patients at higher risk. The rationale for considering selective screening for melanoma is the disproportionate incidence in young adults (18% of melanomas present in people aged 20–35 years compared with

only 4% of all cancers combined in this age group) and the curative potential of early treatment. Studies of the application of melanoma risk scoring systems have suggested that it is possible for patients to self-assess, with reasonable agreement between how patients appraise their skin characteristics compared with physician assessment. This identifies higher risk individuals with the potential to target screening more effectively.

Skin self-examination

Skin self-examination deserves specific mention (Fig. 3.2). Fifty to sixty per cent of melanomas are first identified as being abnormal by patients, 10–20% by spouses or relatives and the remainder by healthcare workers. An American case–control study has suggested that patients who perform skin self-examination present with thinner tumours and consequently have lower mortality rates from melanoma by as much as 63% compared with those who do not perform skin self-examination. More recent data have shown that among melanoma patients who develop a further primary melanoma, those who perform skin self-examination present with thinner tumours than those who do not. Although skin self-examination has not been publicized as much as breast or testicular self-examination, there appears to be sufficient evidence to encourage this in individuals at high risk of skin cancer and in patients who have been diagnosed with a skin cancer.

Referral of suspicious lesions

Access to specialist skin cancer screening clinics is ideally supported by a structured referral letter that enables general practitioners to refer patients whose skin lesions fall within the guidelines for referral. This is important, as data show that, despite the introduction of the '2-week wait' rule for cancer in the UK, many referral letters suggest diagnoses outside the guidelines, do not report diagnoses at all, or do not indicate priority.

New technologies may provide improved triage of patients with suspicious skin lesions. For example, the use of telemedicine providing a live video link to clinics can improve the appropriateness of referring patients to specialist clinics. This is likely to be most useful where geographic access to specialist clinics is poor. Newer technologies include image analysis, but their value and accuracy in early diagnosis are unclear.

- Become familiar with your birthmarks, blemishes and moles so you know what they look like and can detect changes.
- Get undressed. Either use a mirror or the help of a partner for the areas that you cannot see. A suggested scheme is presented below.
- Look at your skin like you look at your watch – a quick first impression is the most valuable assessment.
- Look for new marks, and changes in the size, shape and colour of existing marks. Also look for sores that will not heal, and any growths that may be pink, red, shiny or hard.
- Many skin marks are due to temporary changes. An inflamed spot is a good example – this will settle in 2–3 weeks. A spot lasting >6 weeks needs diagnosing, since it is not showing signs of going away.
- Do this every 2 months.
- Report any marks you are concerned about.

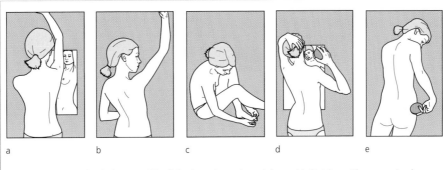

a. Examine your body front and back in the mirror, then right and left sides with arms raised.
b. Bend elbows and look carefully at forearms, upper underarms and palms.
c. Look at the backs of your legs and feet, the spaces between your toes and on the sole.
d. Examine the backs of your neck and scalp with a hand mirror. Part hair for a closer look.
e. Finally, check your back and buttocks with a hand mirror.

Fig. 3.2 Skin self-examination. Patients who perform skin self-examination present with better prognosis thinner melanoma than those who do not. (Figures reprinted with permission from the American Academy of Dermatology.)

Table 3.1 Frequency of follow-up of patients with skin cancer. Follow-up may be based entirely in secondary care or shared with primary care. All patients should be encouraged to self-examine between follow-up appointments and after discharge.

	Recommended frequency of follow-up
BCC	Not usually followed up – patient should be recommended life-long self-examination
SCC	Three to six-monthly for up to 5 years if high risk
Melanoma	Three-monthly for 3 years (plus 6-monthly for a further 2 years if >1 mm in Breslow thickness) – NB This guidance is under review in the UK

Box 3.5 **Useful websites**

For patients:
- British Association of Dermatologists: www.bad.org.uk/public/leaflets/skin-cancer.asp
- Cancer Research UK: www.cancerresearchuk.org
- Cancerbackup: http://www.cancerbackup.org.uk/
- Patient UK: www.patient.co.uk

Health professionals:
- British Association of Dermatologists: www.bad.org.uk/healthcare/guidelines
- Dermnet NZ: www.dermnetnz.org
- E-medicine: www.emedicine.com

Follow-up of patients with skin cancer

Follow-up of patients with skin cancer (Table 3.1) may be based entirely in secondary care or shared with primary care, depending on local arrangements. The most important roles of primary care in following up patients with skin cancer are to ensure that the patient fully understands the nature of the disease and prognosis, how to self-examine for recurrence and for new lesions, and how to reduce the risk of new lesions. This may be reinforced by directing patients to appropriate internet resources (Box 3.5). Supporting patients who are undergoing treatment for skin cancer is also an important role.

Patients who have had a skin cancer should be encouraged to regularly self-examine for local recurrence and new lesions. In cases of SCC and melanoma, patients should also check for recurrences in the surrounding skin and regional lymph nodes (Box 3.6). This is because early detection of recurrent disease may reduce the morbidity and increase the potential for cure from subsequent treatment. Self-examination should be demonstrated by the doctor and preferably performed every 2 months. This involves looking and feeling the skin at the site of the treated tumour, the surrounding skin and the regional lymph nodes. Any new lumps, thickening or ulceration should be reported.

Box 3.6 **Self-examination for recurrence. This should be demonstrated to patients who have had skin cancer**

For all patients:
- Look and feel the treated area for any growths that resemble the original tumour, sores that will not heal, any thickening under the skin, and any other new lumps
- Perform a skin self-examination (see Fig. 3.2)
- Perform this every 2 months
- Report any abnormalities

For patients who have had melanoma or squamous cell carcinoma:
- Additionally, look and feel the skin between the site that was treated and the lymph glands for any growths that resemble the original tumour, sores that won't heal, any thickening under the skin, and any other new lumps
- Feel the glands for any lumps

Further reading

Berwick M, Begg CM, Fine JA *et al.* Screening for cutaneous melanoma by skin self-examination. J Natl Cancer Inst 1996; 88:17–23.

Glazebrook C, Garrud P, Avery A, Coupland C, Williams H. Impact of a multimedia intervention 'skin safe' on patients' knowledge and protective behaviours. Prevent Med 2006; 42:449–54.

MacKie RM, Freudenberger T, Aichinson TC. Personal risk factor chart for cutaneous malignant melanoma. Lancet 1989; 2:487–90.

Montagu M, Borland R, Sinclair C. Slip! Slop! Slap! And Sun Smart 1980–2000: skin cancer control and twenty years of population-based campaigning. Health Educ Behav 2001; 28:290–305.

National Institute for Health and Clinical Excellence (2006). Improving outcomes for people with skin tumours including melanoma. London: National Institute for Clinical Excellence. Available at www.nice.org.uk

Nicholls S. Effect of a public campaign about malignant melanoma on general practitioner workload in Southampton. BMJ 1988; 296:1526–7.

CHAPTER 4

Pre-cancerous skin lesions

Dev Shah, Richard Motley

OVERVIEW

- Premalignant skin lesions include actinic keratosis (AK), Bowen's disease (BD) and lentigo maligna. They are caused by excessive exposure to ultraviolet radiation.

- AK and BD are objective markers of solar damage and do not always require treatment as the rate of transformation to invasive squamous cell carcinoma (SCC) is low.

- The development of induration, nodularity, pain, bleeding and ulceration in AK or BD suggests progression to invasive SCC.

- Providing the diagnosis is certain, AK and BD can be treated in primary care by doctors who are familiar with the treatment options. Lesions that are unresponsive to a single mode of therapy or have developed signs of progression to SCC should be referred to a dermatologist.

- For AK, lesion-directed therapy is indicated if there are few lesions, whereas field-directed therapy is more appropriate if there are many lesions.

- Small BD lesions are treated with cryotherapy or curettage.

- Lentigo maligna can progress to lentigo maligna melanoma and should always be treated, preferably by surgical excision.

- Sun protection and skin self-examination should be encouraged in all patients with premalignant skin lesions.

There are three main pre-cancerous lesions of the skin: actinic keratosis (AK) and Bowen's disease (BD), which may progress to squamous cell carcinoma (SCC), and lentigo maligna (LM), which may progress to lentigo maligna melanoma (LMM). These lesions are caused by excessive cumulative exposure to ultraviolet (UV) radiation in susceptible individuals, typically those with fair skin and light-coloured eyes. The rate at which individual AK and BD lesions transform to SCC is thought to be low. Their presence in large numbers is a warning that the patient has substantial UV-induced skin damage and is at high risk of future SCC, arising from premalignant lesions or *de novo*. Other markers of excessive sun exposure include solar elastosis (yellowish coarse skin), solar lentigines (Fig. 8.2) and seborrhoeic keratoses (Fig. 8.9).

In situ vs. invasive cancer

The skin is comprised of an outer epidermis and an inner dermis, separated by the basement membrane at the dermo-epidermal junction. Epidermal keratinocytes multiply in the basal layer and differentiate as they migrate upwards to form the protective stratum corneum, which is eventually shed. This process takes approximately 30 days. Keratinocytes may acquire UV-induced genetic aberrations leading to abnormal differentiation that can be recognized histologically as dysplasia and clinically as AK and BD (Fig. 4.1). As abnormal cells are limited to the epidermis, these lesions are described as being '*in situ*' SCC. With the accumulation of further genetic mutations, cells may breach the basement membrane, enter the dermis and gain the capacity to metastasize through dermal blood and lymphatic vessels. Lesions at this stage are frankly malignant or 'invasive' SCC. It is important to appreciate that invasive SCC frequently develops *de novo* without going through a clinically recognizable *in situ* phase. Similarly, lentigo maligna is a type of *in situ* melanoma that is confined to the epidermis. Melanoma develops when malignant cells breach the basement membrane and invade the dermis.

Actinic keratosis

In the UK approximately 20% of fair-skinned individuals > 60 years old have one or more AKs, compared with 40–60% of Australians

Fig. 4.1 Progression of premalignant lesions to squamous cell carcinoma (SCC). (a) Actinic keratosis. Dysplastic keratinocytes (shown in red) located in the lower epidermis. (b) Bowen's disease. Dysplastic cells occupy the whole epidermis. (c) Invasive SCC arising within Bowen's disease. Dysplastic keratinocytes have breached the dermo-epidermal junction and invaded the dermis. It is important to appreciate that invasive SCC frequently develops *de novo* without going through a clinically recognizable *in situ* phase.

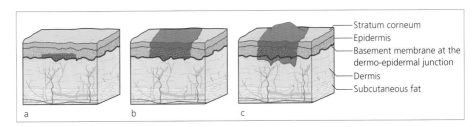

Stratum corneum
Epidermis
Basement membrane at the dermo-epidermal junction
Dermis
Subcutaneous fat

Fig. 4.2 Thin actinic keratosis (AK). There is erythema with minimal scale. On palpation, lesions have a rough texture. Sometimes thin AK is easier to feel than see.

over 40. The risk factors and body site distribution of AK are similar to those of SCC, with a male preponderance and a tendency to occur on exposed sites such as the face, balding scalp, forearms and dorsum of the hands. Small prospective studies have estimated the rate of progression of an individual AK to SCC to be < 0.1 to 0.24% per year. However, up to 25% of untreated AKs may spontaneously regress within a year.

Clinical features

The clinical appearance may vary depending on the amount of scale, from thin superficial AKs, which are rough erythematous patches with only slight scale (Fig. 4.2), to hyperkeratotic AKs, which are papules and plaques with significant adherent scale that may organize to form a keratin horn (Fig. 4.3). The distinction is important, as hyperkeratotic AK may be difficult to distinguish clinically from early SCC, and dense keratin reduces efficacy of topical treatments and liquid nitrogen by impairing penetration. Lesions are usually asymptomatic, but may occasionally itch or be sore.

Investigations

The diagnosis of AK is usually based on the clinical features. Surrounding solar damage in the form of solar lentigines and solar elastosis is usually present. Biopsy to exclude SCC is essential for lesions that are painful, indurated, inflamed or unresponsive to treatment (as these suggest invasive transformation may have occurred) and for hyperkeratotic AKs that cannot be clinically distinguished from SCC.

Treatment

The decision to treat and the choice of treatment is dependent on the individual patient and the type, number and distribution of AKs (Table 4.1). Active treatment is not always necessary, but is warranted if lesions are symptomatic or cosmetically troublesome. There

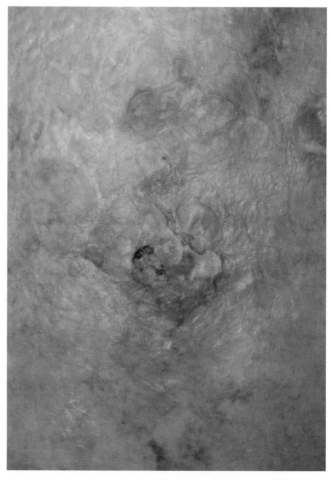

Fig. 4.3 Hyperkeratotic actinic keratoses on the scalp. There is significant adherent yellow-brown scale on these plaques which extend over several centimetres. A wide area of solar damage is often referred to as an area of 'field change'. Note the solar lentigines inferiorly.

Table 4.1 Summary of treatments for actinic keratoses

	Cryosurgery	Curettage	5-Fluorouracil cream	Imiquimod cream	Diclofenac gel	Photodynamic therapy
Number of lesions						
Few (e.g up to 15)	✓✓	✓	✓✓	✓	✓	✓
Many (or area of field change)	✓	✓	✓✓	✓	✓✓	✓✓
Thickness						
Thin	✓✓	–	✓✓	✓	✓✓	✓
Thick (hypertrophic)	–	✓✓	–	–	–	–

✓ ✓, Preferred initial treatment; ✓, suitable alternative treatment; –, unsuitable or rarely used.

are two broad therapeutic approaches: lesion-directed therapy (if there are a few lesions, e.g. < 10 or 15) and field-directed therapy (if lesions are multiple or confluent within a single anatomical area, e.g. the scalp).

Liquid nitrogen cryotherapy is the treatment of choice for lesion-directed therapy, as it is quick and effective, with clearance rates of 70–80% (Fig. 4.4). Curettage and cautery is more effective for hypertrophic AKs and for lesions failing to respond to other interventions. Field-directed therapy involves the use of a topical agent to treat multiple AKs over a wide area of field change. This approach has the added advantage of treating subclinical lesions which are too subtle to see with the naked eye and only become apparent because of the inflammatory reaction from topical agents. In the UK, two topical agents are licensed for the treatment of thin AK–5-fluorouracil cream and diclofenac gel. 5-Fluorouracil cream is more effective, with clearance rates of 70–90%, but often causes a vigorous inflammatory reaction (Fig. 4.5). Diclofenac gel (3%) is better tolerated but less effective. Imiquimod is also effective, but is more expensive and not currently licensed for AK in the UK. Photodynamic therapy (PDT) is used in specialist centres for multiple and confluent lesions in large areas of field change that have not responded to other therapies. Sun avoidance with protective clothing and regular use of sunscreens should be encouraged in all patients, as this may promote regression of existing lesions and reduce the development of further ones.

Follow-up

Adequacy of treatment should be assessed at 8–12 weeks. Those who are unresponsive or have developed signs of progression to SCC should be referred to a dermatologist. Regular follow-up of patients with multiple or confluent AK and of patients who are immunosuppressed can be considered because of the increased risk of skin cancer. Advice on skin self-examination (Fig. 3.2) should be provided to all patients with AKs.

Other keratoses

When AKs occur on the lips, they are known as actinic cheilitis. The lower lip, which receives higher doses of UV radiation, may become scaly, develop greyish white plaques and become smooth from loss of skin lines and blunting of the vermillion border (Fig. 4.6). Actinic

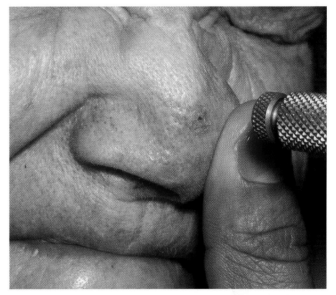

(a)

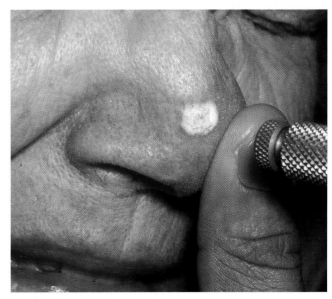

(b)

Fig. 4.4 Lesion-directed therapy of an actinic keratosis with liquid nitrogen cryotherapy. The lesion and 1–2 mm of surrounding skin are treated for 5–10 s.

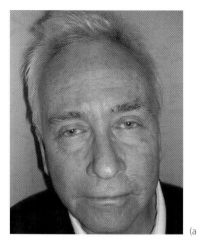 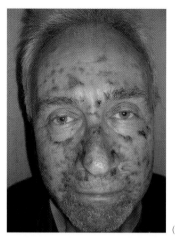 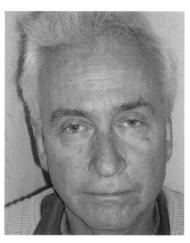

Fig. 4.5 Field-directed therapy for multiple actinic keratoses (AKs) on the face with 5-fluorouracil cream twice daily for 4 weeks. (a) Before treatment. (b) An aggressive inflammatory reaction and secondary impetiginization is evident at the end of the 4-week treatment period. Subclinical lesions also become apparent. (c) There are significantly fewer AKs at 3 months follow-up.

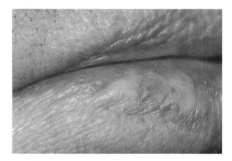

Fig. 4.6 Actinic cheilitis. There are grey-white patches on the lower lip, loss of skin lines and blunting of the lower vermilion border.

cheilitis probably carries a greater risk of progression to SCC, which may manifest as a nodule, fissure or ulcer (Fig. 5.4). Actinic cheilitis should be referred to a specialist for treatment with cryotherapy, 5-fluorouracil cream, laser ablation or vermilionectomy.

Bowen's disease

The annual incidence of BD may be as high as 15 per 100 000 in the UK. Like AK, BD is also caused by solar damage. However, BD has a distinct female preponderance (with a 3 : 1 female to male ratio) and a tendency to affect the lower legs disproportionately more than other exposed areas. The risk of progression to SCC is estimated to be as high as 3% per year.

Clinical features

BD presents as a fixed, gradually enlarging, well-demarcated, erythematous, scaly plaque (Fig. 4.7). Lesions are usually solitary, but may be multiple in 20% of patients. Lesions may be difficult to distinguish from superficial basal cell carcinoma (BCC) (Fig. 7.12). Rare variants include the verrucous form, which simulates viral warts, and the pigmented form, which may be confused with melanoma.

Investigations

The diagnosis of BD is usually based on the clinical features, although a biopsy may be required to differentiate lesions from AK and superficial BCC. As with AK, invasive transformation is likely if

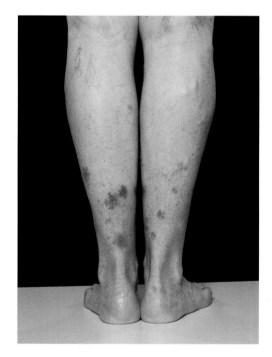

(a)

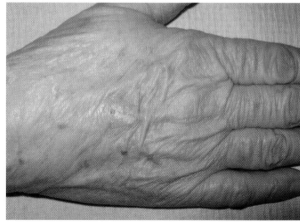

(b)

Fig. 4.7 (a) Multiple lesions of Bowen's disease (BD) on the lower leg of an older female. Seventy per cent of BD is found on the lower legs. (b) Close up view of a lesion on the dorsum of the hand.

Table 4.2 Summary of treatments for Bowen's disease

	Cryotherapy	Curettage	5-Fluorouracil cream	Imiquimod cream	Photodynamic therapy	Excision
Good healing site						
Small and few lesions	✓✓	✓✓	✓	✓	✓	✓
Large and few, or multiple lesions	✓	✓	✓✓	✓	✓✓	✓
Poor healing site, e.g. below the knee, flexures, ears	–	–	✓✓	✓	✓✓	–

✓✓, Preferred initial treatment; ✓, suitable alternative treatment; –, unsuitable, rarely used or used cautiously.

lesions are repeatedly unresponsive to treatment or become painful, indurated (Fig. 5.6), nodular, inflamed or ulcerated (Fig. 7.13).

Treatment

Cryotherapy or curettage and cautery are usually considered first-line treatments for smaller lesions (Table 4.2). Both these approaches destroy tissue and create an area of ulceration that is left to heal by secondary intention. Destructive therapies for larger or multiple lesions in poor healing sites such as the lower legs should be used with caution, as healing is significantly slower. 5-Fluorouracil cream, PDT or simple observation may be preferred in these circumstances. Overall, 10–20% of treated lesions recur.

Follow-up

A similar approach to follow-up for AK can be adopted.

Other *in situ* SCC

In situ SCC can uncommonly occur in the anogenital area. Lesions developing on the glans penis in older uncircumcised men are known as erythroplasia of Queyrat (Fig. 4.8) and carry a 10% risk of progression to SCC. This condition can be mistaken for balanitis. However, balanitis tends to fluctuate, whereas *in situ* SCC is fixed. Bowenoid papulosis is another form of genital *in situ* SCC that occurs as discrete papules on the penile shaft or vulva of younger individuals, and has a lower tendency to progress to SCC. Infection with human papillomavirus types 16 and 18 is believed to have a pathogenic role for genital *in situ* SCC.

Lentigo maligna

Lentigo maligna is a pre-cancerous neoplasm in which malignant melanocytes are restricted to the epidermis. It develops on chronically sun-exposed skin as a slowly enlarging, irregularly pigmented macule (Fig. 4.9) that can sometimes be hard to distinguish from a solar lentigo. Treatment is required, as 5–15% of lesions progress to LMM, which occurs when malignant melanocytes breach the basement membrane causing the lesion to become raised, darker and nodular. Surgical excision is the treatment of choice for lentigo ma-

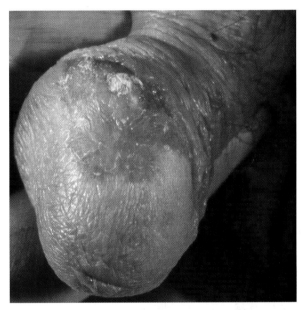

Fig. 4.8 Erythroplasia de Queyrat. There is a fixed plaque on the glans penis in this elderly uncircumcised patient that was treated as balanitis for several months despite the absence of inflammation.

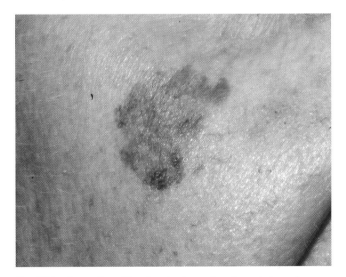

Fig. 4.9 Lentigo maligna. There is a slowly growing pigmented macule, which is irregular in colour and outline.

ligna, although radiotherapy is an effective alternative for situations where surgery is contraindicated.

Further reading

Berman B, Bienstock L, Kuritzky L *et al*. Actinic keratoses: sequelae and treatments. Recommendations from a consensus panel. J Family Pract 2006; May Supplement:1–8.

Cox NH, Eedy DJ, Morton CA; on behalf of the British Association of Dermatologists Therapy Guidelines and Audit Subcommittee. Guidelines for management of Bowen's disease: 2006 update. Br J Dermatol 2007; 156:11–21.

de Berker D, McGregor JM, Hughes BR; on behalf of the British Association of Dermatologists Therapy Guidelines and Audit Subcommittee. Guidelines for the management of actinic keratoses. Br J Dermatol 2007; 156:222–30.

CHAPTER 5

Squamous cell carcinoma

Sajjad Rajpar, Jerry Marsden

OVERVIEW

- Squamous cell carcinomas (SCCs) can grow rapidly over weeks to months, and have the capacity to metastasize.
- Most SCCs are nodules, although some are ulcers. SCC should be excluded in any non-healing ulcer.
- Induration is an important physical sign of SCC.
- Surgical excision is treatment of choice for SCC.
- Five-year survival is almost 100% for low-risk SCC and 70% for high-risk SCC.
- Keratoacanthomas can be difficult to distinguish from SCC, and are best managed by excision as for SCC.
- Secondary prevention is important, and photoprotection should be encouraged in patients who have had a solar-induced SCC.

Box 5.1 **Key points in the history**

- Duration – usually 4 weeks to 6 months
- Rate of growth – poorer prognosis if rapid
- Symptoms such as bleeding and pain are indicative of dermal invasion
- Preceding lesion at same site, e.g. actinic keratosis, Bowen's disease, scar, ulcer, chronic inflammation
- Previously treated squamous cell carcinoma at same site – suggests recurrence
- Presence of other risk factors

Squamous cell carcinoma (SCC) is the second most common cutaneous malignancy. It may arise *de novo* or from pre-cancerous lesions such as actinic keratosis (AK) and Bowen's disease. Cumulative exposure to ultraviolet (UV) radiation is the leading cause, hence the majority of lesions are seen on sun-exposed sites in patients who have fair skin and are > 60 years old. Seventy to 80% of SCCs occur on the head and neck, especially the lower lip, ears and scalp. Other common sites are the dorsal surfaces of the hands, forearms and lower legs. SCC on non-exposed skin does occur, but is much less common. Patients who are immunosuppressed after an organ transplant are estimated to be at a 65–250-fold greater risk of developing SCC. Other risk factors are discussed in Chapter 2.

History

SCCs are recognized by patients as growths that have developed over a period of several weeks or months (Box 5.1). Keratoacanthomas (KAs) develop at a similar rate and cannot be distinguished by the history alone. Lesions are usually asymptomatic, but may be tender. Bleeding often occurs because SCCs invade dermal blood vessels. KAs are epidermal lesions that do not invade the dermis and so do not normally bleed, a useful clinical distinction.

Clinical appearance

Most SCCs are ulcerated nodules, although some present as expand-ing ulceration and others as plaques. A consistent physical sign in SCC is induration, which is thickening at the edge or base of a lesion that represents infiltration of the dermis by tumour cells. Induration is not a feature of benign and premalignant epidermal lesions. When SCC occurs on sun-exposed sites, surrounding solar damage, including solar lentigines and AK, is often present. SCC occurring in immunosuppressed patients tends to be more aggressive and yet can appear deceptively banal.

Nodules

Most SCCs begin as skin-coloured to erythematous papules and plaques that develop into nodules (Fig. 5.1). Lesions display differing degrees of keratinization, which is a feature of better differentiated tumours and manifests as the presence of scale, a cen-

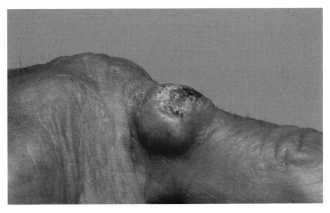

Fig. 5.1 Squamous cell carcinoma. There is an erythematous infiltrated nodule with scale and crust concealing a centrally ulcerated area.

tral keratin plug or a keratin horn. Fifteen per cent of all keratin horns arise from an SCC (Fig. 5.2). Ulceration usually occurs as lesions increase in size, giving a pink, infiltrated, raised edge that may be mistaken for the pearly rolled edge of a nodulo-ulcerative basal cell carcinoma (BCC). Poorly differentiated tumours do not keratinize much, appearing as eroded and friable erythematous nodules (Fig. 5.3). Exudate and fibrin may form a crust at sites of ulceration, occasionally concealing infection and pus. This should be carefully removed to permit better visualization of the lesion. Advanced tumours may invade so deeply that they become fixed to deeper structures.

Ulcers

SCC can present as an ulcer (Fig. 5.4). The edge is irregular, indurated and usually everted, whereas the base is erythematous and friable. This appearance is more common on the scalp of balding men, lower legs, and in Marjolin's ulcers (SCC that arises in long-standing scars and benign ulcers). SCC complicates 0.2% of venous leg ulcers, but may also masquerade as a venous leg ulcer (Fig. 5.5). Warning clues include the presence of an isolated expanding ulcer

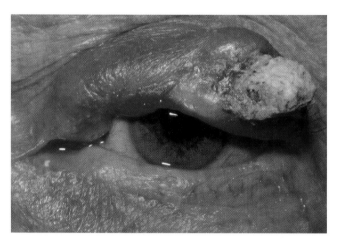

Fig. 5.2 Keratin horn arising from a squamous cell carcinoma (SCC). The base of this keratin horn is extensively indurated, suggesting the lesion is an SCC. Other causes of a keratin horn include actinic keratosis, Bowen's disease, viral wart and seborrhoeic keratosis – the base in these lesions would not be indurated.

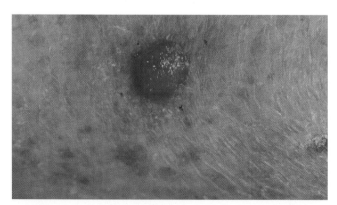

Fig. 5.3 Poorly differentiated squamous cell carcinoma. There is an eroded erythematous nodule with surrounding erythema that reflects induration and spread.

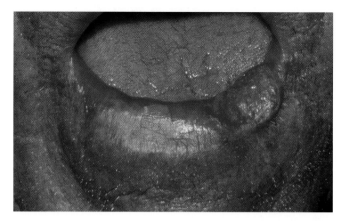

Fig. 5.4 Ulcerative squamous cell carcinoma. There is a malignant ulcer with everted and indurated edges.

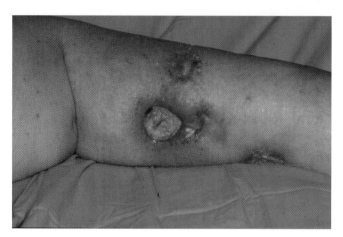

Fig. 5.5 Ulcerative squamous cell carcinoma. This lesion was treated as a venous leg ulcer. However, it is above the gaiter area and lacks surrounding features of venous hypertension.

that is refractory to treatment and the absence of venous hypertensive changes in the surrounding skin (Box 5.2). It is important to be aware that SCC can mimic or complicate benign lesions in this way, as diagnosis is often delayed.

Plaques

Thickening and induration in a patch or plaque of AK or Bowen's disease suggests transformation to SCC. The presence of pain, bleeding, ulceration and persistent lack of response to treatments in these lesions should also alert to the possibility of invasive transformation (Fig. 5.6).

Box 5.2 **Features suggestive of malignancy in an ulcer**

- Chronic duration (> 3 months)
- No apparent cause
- Everted, indurated or ill-defined edges
- Developed in a long-standing scar or area of chronic inflammation
- Unresponsive to treatment
- Increasing in size despite treatment
- Repeated ulceration after apparent healing

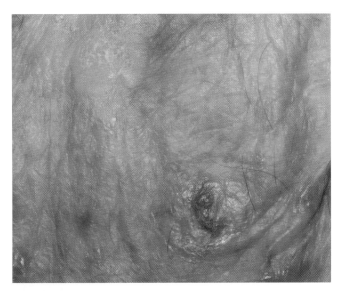

Fig. 5.6 Induration (thickening) and superficial ulceration in a Bowen's disease lesion. Histology confirmed transformation to squamous cell carcinoma had occurred.

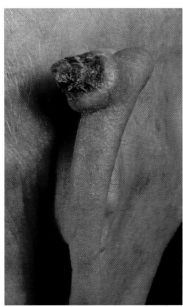

Fig. 5.7 Keratoacanthoma. There is an erythematous nodule with a central keratin plug which is indistinguishable from a well-differentiated squamous cell carcinoma.

As it is not always possible to determine early invasive transformation clinically, biopsy may be required. If the clinical signs strongly suggest SCC, it may be better to excise the whole lesion for accurate diagnosis, avoiding misdiagnosis due to biopsy sampling error.

Rare clinical types

Verrucous SCC resembles viral warts. They may occur on the soles, around nails and in the anogenital region. Although uncommon, this diagnosis should be considered in non-resolving and atypical warts in those > 40 years old.

Keratoacanthoma

It is uncertain whether KA is a well-differentiated and self-limiting variant of SCC without the capacity to metastasize, or a separate entity. Lesions arise from normal skin as dome-shaped growths with a central keratin plug (Fig. 5.7). They usually attain a size of 1–3 cm within 4–6 weeks, then spontaneously involute over 6–10 weeks, leaving a depressed atrophic scar. KAs tend to arise on sun-exposed skin with the same preponderance for age and skin type as SCC. Lesions can be locally destructive and 5% recur after excision

For practical purposes, a lesion that has the history and appearance of an isolated KA is probably best managed as an SCC with surgical excision and histological analysis. This is because the history, physical signs and biopsy findings of KA are not easily distinguished from well-differentiated SCC, particularly as there are no universally accepted histological criteria separating the two. Although spontaneous resolution of KA may occur before treatment, awaiting spontaneous involution generates anxiety, can occasionally lead to significant tissue destruction, may result in cosmetically prominent scarring, and runs the risk of significant progression in those lesions which are actually SCC rather than KA.

Initial management

Once the diagnosis of SCC is suspected, the regional lymph nodes should be palpated for metastases and the rest of the skin should be examined for other skin malignancies. In the UK, urgent referral to a secondary care-based skin oncology service should be made under the 2-week wait rule, as SCC can grow rapidly. Biopsy in primary care cannot be recommended as false-negative results are not infrequent, and resultant treatment delay may seriously worsen outcome.

Treatment

Surgery

Surgical excision is the treatment of choice for SCC (Box 5.3), as it enables histological confirmation of the diagnosis and assessment of resection margins to ensure completeness of excision. Full-thickness excision of the skin and the whole subcutaneous layer is performed. As for BCC, a margin of surrounding uninvolved skin is also ex-

---

Box 5.3 **Summary of treatment options for squamous cell carcinoma**

Surgery
- Standard excision with wide margins (treatment of choice)
- Mohs' micrographic surgery

Radiotherapy

Others (only suitable for small (<6 mm in diameter) low-risk squamous cell carcinoma)
- Curettage and cautery
- Cryosurgery

---

cised to ensure any subclinical cancerous spread is not left behind. The minimum margin size required to ensure at least 95% chance of complete excision is 6 mm and increases with tumour diameter. The majority of surgical defects can be closed directly, although a local flap or skin graft may be required. Most surgery is performed under local anaesthetic as a day case procedure.

Radiotherapy

Radiotherapy produces cure rates of >90%, which are broadly similar to those achieved with surgery. It is particularly useful for sites where surgical reconstruction may be difficult, and for treating patients who are unfit for an operation. However, radiotherapy can further injure solar-damaged skin, and adds the risk of radiation-induced cancer to already cancer-prone skin. To minimize secondary cancer risk, its use is limited to those >60–65 years old.

Curettage and cautery/cryotherapy

These modalities can be used to treat low-risk tumours – those that are ≤6 mm in diameter and do not have any of the features associated with an increased risk of local recurrence or metastasis described below. However, surgical excision is preferable, as these techniques do not permit histological analysis of margins or of tumour thickness, are highly operator dependent and require careful patient selection. Use of these modalities should therefore be reserved for experienced clinicians.

Complications and prognosis

Local spread can lead to bleeding and secondary infection and, eventually, deeper destruction of muscle and bone. Pain and neuropathy may occur if nerves have been infiltrated. The overall 5-year survival rate is almost 100% for low-risk SCC, and 70% for those with multiple high-risk features (Table 5.1). In the first 5 years after treatment, 8% of tumours recur locally and 3–5% metastasize. Predicting the exact risk of recurrence or metastasis for an individual lesion is difficult because large studies assessing the individual contribution of prognostic factors by multivariate analysis are lacking. When metastases occur, 85% develop in the regional lymph nodes, with a 5-year survival of 30%. Haematogenous spread to solid organs and the skeleton is less common and carries a 5-year survival of < 10%.

Follow-up

There are no studies evaluating the value of following up patients with SCC, though three-quarters of local recurrences and metastases occur within 2 years of diagnosis, and almost half develop a further cutaneous malignancy. It seems sensible to observe patients regularly for the development of these eventualities, as timely detection may better enable curative intervention. In the UK, it is recommended that patients with high-risk SCC (> 1 cm in diameter, rapidly growing or poorly differentiated) are followed up for a period of 5 years. However, the frequency of follow-up visits, whether they are undertaken in primary or secondary care, and follow-up for low-risk SCC are highly variable and often decided locally. Patient education and encouragement of life-long self-examination form an essential part of follow-up.

Further reading

Alam D, Ratner D. Cutaneous squamous-cell carcinoma. N Engl J Med 2001; 344:975–83.

Motley R, Kersey P, Lawrence C. Multiprofessional guidelines for the management of the patient with primary cutaneous squamous cell carcinoma. Br J Dermatol 2002; 146:18–25.

National comprehensive cancer network. Clinical practice guidelines in Oncology. Basal cell and squamous cell skin cancers v2.2005. Available at www.nccn.org/professionals/physician_gls/PDF/nmsc.pdf

Schwartz R. Keratoacanthoma: a clinico-pathologic enigma. Dermatol Surg 2004; 30:326–33.

Table 5.1 High-risk features in SCC

	Relative risk of local recurrence	Relative risk of metastasis
Clinical features		
Greater than 2 cm in diameter	2	3
Located on the eyelid, ear, nose, lip, scalp, anogenital	2–3	2–3
Marjolin ulcer	–	5
Rapid growth	–	–
Recurrent SCC	3	4
Histological features		
Greater than 4 mm deep or Clark level 5 (reaches subcutaneous fat)	2	5
Poorly differentiated/spindle cell/desmoplastic	2	3
Perineural invasion	5	5
Patient features		
Immunosuppression	–	2
Chronic lymphocytic leukaemia	–	3–4

The presence of these features is associated with an increased risk of local recurrence and metastases.
SCC, Squamous cell carcinoma.

CHAPTER 6

Basal cell carcinoma

Sajjad Rajpar, Jerry Marsden

OVERVIEW

- Basal cell carcinomas (BCCs) are slow growing and develop over months to several years. They invade local tissues but hardly ever metastasize.

- A translucent pink colour and multiple surface telangiectasias are important physical signs of BCC.

- Most BCCs are nodular. Morphoeic BCC is the most subtle variant and can mimic a scar.

- Surgical excision is the treatment of choice for BCC. Radiotherapy is a suitable alternative for situations where surgical excision is contraindicated.

- A variety of non-surgical treatments have become available for superficial BCC, including topical chemotherapy, topical immunotherapy and photodynamic therapy.

- Thirty to 40% of patients develop another BCC within 5 years. Skin self-examination and photoprotection should therefore be encouraged.

Basal cell carcinoma (BCC) is the most common malignancy in White populations, accounting for 75% of skin cancers. Metastatic spread and death are exceedingly rare, but local tissue destruction occurs insidiously and can be extensive. Most BCCs develop on the face, followed by the trunk and extremities (Table 6.1). Unlike squamous cell carcinomas (SCCs), they never occur on the palms, soles or mucous membranes. The majority of lesions fall into one of three distinct clinical and histological subtypes: nodular, superficial and morphoeic. The presence of overlapping features within a single lesion is well recognized. Two further histological patterns of growth, micronodular and infiltrative, may coexist in any subtype. Ultraviolet (UV) radiation is the main causal factor, and the typical susceptible phenotype has fair skin and red or blond hair. Intermittent high-intensity UV exposure during the first two decades of life may be more important than cumulative lifetime exposure. Aetiology and risk factors are discussed further in Chapter 2.

History

BCCs typically start developing after the age of 60 years, although they are increasingly seen in younger adults. They are slower growing than SCCs, and develop over a period of months to several years (Box 6.1). Most lesions are asymptomatic and many eventually ulcerate. Ulceration may be intermittent at first, leading to periodic bleeding.

Clinical appearance

Useful diagnostic characteristics of BCC are a shiny or translucent pink colour and the presence of multiple surface telangiectasias. Gently stretching the skin, removing adherent crust and ensuring there is good oblique illumination makes these signs easier to see. BCCs can usually be diagnosed by their clinical features, although a biopsy is required if there is diagnostic doubt. Ten per cent of patients have more than one BCC at presentation, so it is important to examine the rest of the skin.

Nodular BCC and its variants

Nodular BCC is mainly found on the head and neck. Lesions begin as papules (Fig. 2.2) that grow into nodules which may ulcerate (Fig. 6.1). Asymmetrical growth may produce a multilobulated appearance. Central ulceration in a nodule leaves a raised, rolled edge. These lesions are known as 'rodent ulcers' or nodulo-ulcerative BCCs (Fig. 6.2). Occasionally, a nodular BCC may accumulate mucinous substance giving rise to a cyst. This variant is known as nodulo-cystic BCC (Fig. 6.3).

Table 6.1 Frequency of basal cell carcinoma subtypes at different body sites (%) (adapted from Y. Scrivener *et al.* Br J Dermatol 2002; 147:41–47)

Subtype	Head and neck	Trunk	Extremities	Overall
Nodular (*n* = 9633)	90	6	4	**79**
Superficial (*n* = 1850)	40	46	14	**15**
Morphoeic (*n* = 761)	95	3	2	**6**
Overall	**83**	**12**	**5**	**100**

Box 6.1 **Key points in the history**

- Duration – 3 months at least; several years is common
- Rate of growth – slow growing but variable
- Symptoms – bleeding, scabbing, pain
- Previously treated basal cell carcinoma at same site – suggests recurrence

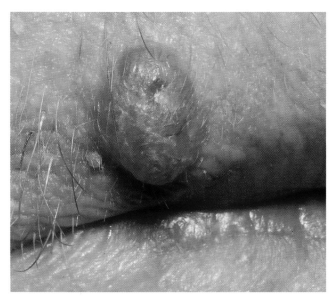

Fig. 6.1 Nodular basal cell carcinoma. There is a translucent ('pearly') pink nodule with several telangiectasias and some adherent crust inferiorly.

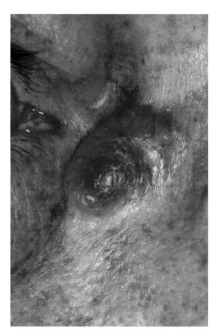

Fig. 6.3 Nodulo-cystic basal cell carcinoma. Mucin accumulation in a nodular BCC leads to the formation of a cyst.

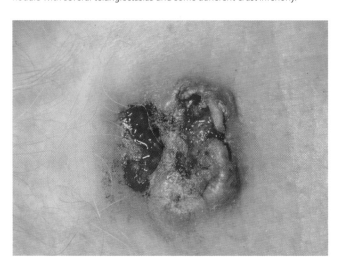

Fig. 6.2 Nodulo-ulcerative basal cell carcinoma ('rodent ulcer'). Central ulceration in a nodular BCC gives rise to a raised, rolled edge.

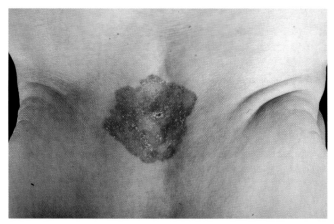

Fig. 6.4 Superficial basal cell carcinoma. There is a well-demarcated pink plaque with raised borders, that has attained a size of several centimetres over almost 10 years.

Superficial BCC

Superficial BCCs occur with equal frequency on the head and neck as on the trunk. Lesions appear as well-demarcated plaques with a characteristic bright pink colour and a thread-like raised pearly border (Fig. 6.4). They are sometimes mistaken for psoriasis, eczema and Bowen's disease. Superficial BCCs do not penetrate very deeply into the skin, but have a tendency to grow outwards and can attain a size of several centimetres. Growth occurs in finger-like projections that may not be visible, leading to seemingly new plaques arising in close proximity to existing ones (Fig. 7.12). These lesions were previously called multifocal BCC, but 3D modelling has demonstrated that individual plaques are frequently interconnected in the dermis and are part of a single lesion.

Morphoeic BCC

Morphoeic BCCs are the least common subtype, and appear as slightly raised or depressed white, grey or yellow scars as a result of a strong fibrotic reaction to neoplastic cells (Fig. 6.5). They are highly invasive, have ill-defined borders and often lack typical features such as erythema and telangiectasias, which can make them difficult to identify. Lesions may therefore spread quite extensively before they are detected.

Pigmented BCC

Overall, 2% of BCCs are pigmented (Fig. 6.6). Any BCC subtype may have a degree of pigmentation, although a raised border, shininess and telangiectasias are usually present and help to make the diagnosis. Pigmented BCC can be confused with melanoma.

Growth and invasion

The growth rate of BCC varies considerably – some lesions grow over several months to several years, others grow in bursts and

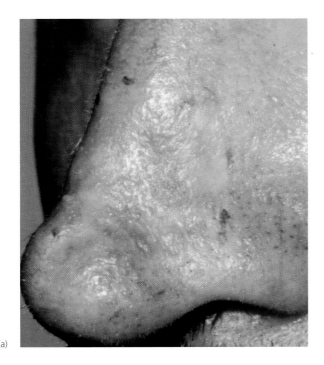

(a)

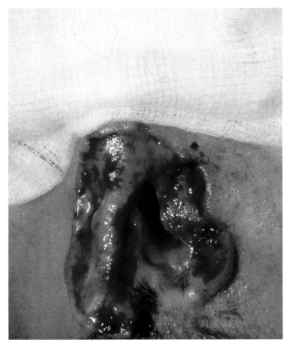

(b)

Fig. 6.5 Morphoeic basal cell carcinoma. (a) There is a scar-like plaque on the nose. Palpation reveals the lesion to be indurated beyond the visible margins. (b) The lesion was treated with Mohs' micrographic excision, showing the extensive invasion that has occurred through the cartilage.

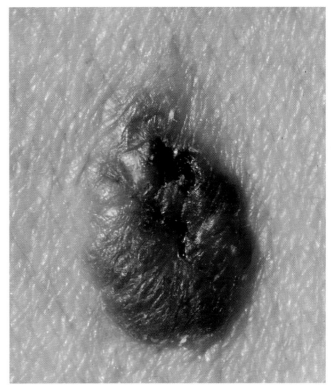

Fig. 6.6 Pigmented basal cell carcinoma. There is a multilobulated pigmented nodule, with a pearlescent superior edge. Clinical differentiation from nodular melanoma is difficult.

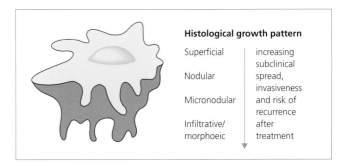

Fig. 6.7 Three-dimensional image of a basal cell carcinoma. Growth occurs by finger-like projections that cannot be seen with the naked eye (red). Subclinical spread, invasiveness and recurrence after treatment vary with histological subtype.

Treatment

It is important to reassure patients that BCC is not life-threatening and can be cured. The goal of treatment is to eliminate the tumour with minimal morbidity and with sparing of uninvolved skin. Failure to eliminate the entire tumour may lead to local recurrence and further invasion of tissue. Recurrences usually develop in the first 3–5 years after treatment. Certain tumour characteristics, in addition to the histological pattern, are associated with an increased risk of recurrence after treatment. Lesions with these features are known as 'high-risk' BCC (Box 6.2).

Despite the huge worldwide burden from BCC, there are surprisingly few good data on treatment. A recent Cochrane review identified 27 randomized controlled trials (RCTs), only three of which

some are apparently static for years. Lesions grow in three dimensions by finger-like projections that infiltrate surrounding tissues (Fig. 6.7). These extensions may be 'subclinical', i.e. not visible to the naked eye, but still need to be adequately treated to prevent continued invasion and recurrence. The histological growth pattern is the best predictor of the degree of subclinical extension, the tendency to invade local structures, and the tendency to recur after treatment.

Box 6.2 **High-risk basal cell carcinoma. The presence of any of these features is associated with an increased risk of recurrence after treatment**

- Location: 'H–zone' of the face (periorbital, eyebrows, nose, perioral, nasolabial folds, pre and post auricular)
- Histology: micronodular, infiltrative or morphoeic
- Borders: ill defined
- Size: > 2 cm in diameter
- Recurrent: previous radiotherapy or surgery
- Immunosuppression

involved surgical excision. Several large case series exist, although significant variability in methodology between studies and the inherent inferior quality of evidence from this type of study design impose limitations. The available evidence shows that surgical excision offers the best chance of cure (Table 6.2). Cure rates with radiotherapy approach those of surgery. Chemical [topical 5-fluorouracil (5-FU)], photochemical (photodynamic therapy) and immunological (imiquimod) treatments are alternative options for superficial BCC. The choice of treatment will rest upon the type, location and size of the BCC, as well as patient factors including age, preference and comorbidity. Clinicians treating BCC must be well versed with the entire therapeutic selection so as to be able to tailor treatments to individual circumstances. In the UK, most lesions located on the head and neck and all high-risk lesions are managed by specialists.

Surgery

Surgical excision is the treatment of choice, as it produces the highest cure rate and enables histological assessment of the tumour. Surgery is usually carried out in the ambulatory care setting under local anaesthesia. A predetermined margin of uninvolved skin around the tumour is also excised in order to include areas of subclinical spread. For example, at least 4 mm must removed around lesions that are up to 2 cm in diameter to give 95% confidence that the tumour is completely excised. Surgical defects are therefore larger than visible tumour dimensions. Large defects may require complex surgical reconstruction. Mohs' micrographic surgery is used in specialist centres for excising difficult high-risk lesions.

Table 6.2 Summary of treatment options for basal cell carcinoma (BCC) and approximate 5-year cure rates. Heterogeneity of studies precludes direct comparison of cure rates between treatment modalities

Intervention	Approximate 5-year cure rates for previously untreated BCC, %
Mohs' micrographic surgery	> 95
Surgical excision	92–97
Radiotherapy	90–95
Cryotherapy	80–90
Curettage and cautery	80–95
5-FU*	75–80
Imiquimod*	75–80
Photodynamic therapy*	70–95

*Rates quoted for superficial BCC only.

Radiotherapy

Cure rates with radiotherapy are high. There is only one RCT comparing radiotherapy with surgical excision (with frozen section analysis), which showed recurrence rates at 4 years of 0.7% in the surgery group compared with 7.5% in the radiotherapy group. Radiotherapy is a useful modality in patients > 65 years old for lesions on the head and neck in instances where surgery is contraindicated or may lead to a poor cosmetic or functional outcome.

Curettage and cautery/cryotherapy

Cure rates with these modalities tend to be lower than with surgery or radiotherapy, and are heavily operator dependent. Both techniques create an ulcer that is left to heal by secondary intention. Healing time is longer and cosmetic results may be inferior compared with surgery. As the perimeter of the tumour is not analysed histologically, it is never certain whether all tumour cells have been removed. These techniques are most suitable for small (< 1 cm) low-risk BCC by experienced operators.

Topical treatment of superficial BCC

Superficial BCCs do not infiltrate deeply into the skin and so are amenable to topical treatments such as 5-FU, imiquimod and photodynamic therapy. Cure rates from these interventions are inferior to those achieved by surgical excision, and data on the long-term recurrence rates are poor. Despite this, topical treatments are useful in situations where there are multiple lesions, or where surgery is undesirable.

Complications and prognosis

If left untreated, BCCs are capable of extensive tissue destruction through nerves, cartilage and bone. Only a small number of lesions that are treated appropriately recur, typically in the first 5 years after treatment. Recurrent BCC is often more aggressive, and is usually treated surgically. Metastasis is exceedingly rare, and reported in fewer than one in 10 000 cases.

Follow-up

Most patients are not followed up after treatment, although almost 30–40% of patients develop further BCC sometime in the future. Patients can be asked to perform regular skin self-examination for local recurrences and new lesions (Box 3.5). This should be supplemented with advice on sun protection.

Further reading

Avril MF, Auperin A, Marqulis A et al. Basal cell carcinoma of the face: surgery or radiotherapy? Results of a randomized study. Br J Cancer 1997; 76:100–6.

Bath-Hextall F, Perkins W, Bong J, Williams H. Interventions for basal cell carcinoma of the skin. Cochrane Database Syst Rev 2007; Issue 1.

Motley RJ, Gould DJ, Douglas WS, Simpson NB. Treatment of basal cell carcinoma by dermatologists in the United Kingdom. British Association of Dermatologists Audit Subcommittee and the British Society for Dermatological Surgery. Br J Dermatol 1995; 132:437–40.

CHAPTER 7

Differential diagnosis of non-melanoma skin cancer

Graham Colver

OVERVIEW

- The appearance of non-melanoma skin cancer (NMSC) can vary because of several factors, including degree of differentiation, anatomical location and presence of surface breakdown.
- Common benign skin lesions may mimic NMSC. The converse is also true, and NMSC may mimic benign skin lesions. Specific features in the history and examination help distinguish the two, although a biopsy is sometimes required.
- Immunosuppressed patients often have clinically atypical skin cancers which can look deceptively benign.
- A low threshold for suspecting malignancy needs to be maintained in certain clinical scenarios such as an expanding red nodule, non-healing ulcers and scaly lower leg lesions.

Non-melanoma skin cancer (NMSC) is a collective term for basal cell carcinoma (BCC) and squamous cell carcinoma (SCC). No attempt is made in this chapter to discuss rare skin cancers. Clinicians who wish to diagnose NMSC must be aware of its range of possible presentations and the varied morphology that can be seen in benign conditions. Essential aids are a bright light, magnification and, more recently, a dermatoscope. The text is divided into three sections:
- Inherent difficulties – variation in presentation
- Lesions that can mimic NMSC
- Specific clinical situations.

Inherent difficulties – variation in presentation

Typical appearance
In 1827 Arthur Jacob wrote his classical description of BCC using terms such as 'destructive ulceration …slowness of progress …edges elevated, smooth and glossy …serpentine outline …healthy looking granulations'. This was an elegant description but only pertinent to the nodulo-ulcerative subtype of BCC. In clinical practice we see scaly lesions, ill-defined plaques, pigmentation and even warty nodules, all having a histological diagnosis of BCC. The textbook description of an SCC describes a firm, pink, fleshy-based lesion with a central core of keratin, but clinically it may be a non-specific eroded patch, a red nodule which may be ulcerated, or keratin growing directly from an apparently normal base.

These variations can be explained by:
- Degree of differentiation of the tumour
- Host immunocompetence
- Anatomical site
- Presence or absence of surface breakdown
- Degrees of pigmentation.

An example of the variations seen in benign lesions is the ubiquitous seborrhoeic keratosis. It may be skin coloured, flat and scaly like a superficial BCC, shiny like a nodulocystic BCC, fast-growing, keratinous and exophytic like a well-differentiated SCC, or inflamed, necrotic and ulcerated as seen in poorly differentiated SCC.

Immunosuppression
Immunosuppressed patients often have clinically atypical skin cancers which can look deceptively benign. A lower threshold of suspicion is required, and this may include biopsying small warty lesions and red patches which might otherwise have been overlooked.

Crust or keratin?
Exudate with fibrin will adhere to an erosion or ulcer to form a nondescript cover. It is essential to remove this crust, by soaking if necessary, to reveal the underlying pathology and facilitate diagnosis (Fig. 7.1). Keratin, in contrast, is part of the epidermis and so cannot be easily removed. If present, it points to a squamopro-

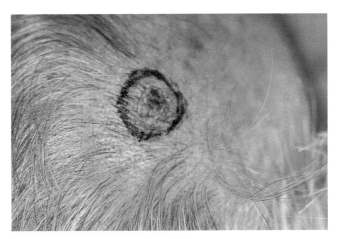

Fig. 7.1 Crust due to exudation from a basal cell carcinoma can usually be removed.

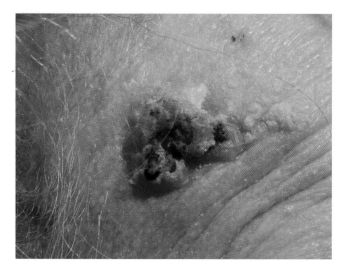

Fig. 7.2 Keratin may cover actinic keratosis, Bowen's disease and well-differentiated squamous cell carcinoma and is not easily removed.

liferative lesion such as Bowen's disease, actinic keratosis (AK) or SCC (Fig. 7.2).

Lesions that can mimic NMSC (Table 7.1)

Actinic keratosis

Typically they have a sandpapery feel, but some variants produce exudate, keratin horns and other features that mimic both BCC and SCC. Rapid growth and induration at the base are suggestive of SCC.

Bowen's disease

It may be impossible to distinguish between Bowen's disease and superficial BCC. This is particularly so on the lower limb, but also on the trunk. There may be a characteristic thread-like edge to a superficial BCC, but otherwise little difference. Both the hyper-

trophic and ulcerated forms of Bowen's can be confused with SCC.

Other skin cancers

Keratoacanthoma is hard to distinguish from invasive SCC, but the characteristic onion shape and very rapid growth favour a diagnosis of keratoacanthoma.

Atypical BCC and SCC can be confused with each other, especially at some sites such as the ear. Melanoma may resemble a pigmented BCC and, in its amelanotic form, SCC. Fast-growing red nodules may represent aggressive skin cancers, and are discussed below.

Sebaceous hyperplasia

These lesions are usually multiple and seen on the forehead, nose and cheeks (Fig. 7.3). Their translucency and telangiectasia may resemble BCC, but the colour is yellow and a tiny central depression is normally seen.

Pyogenic granuloma

This is a red, exophytic nodule that grows over 2–6 weeks (Fig. 7.4). It characteristically bleeds profusely on contact – the absence of this symptom suggests alternative, probably more serious, pathology such as amelanotic nodular melanoma or high-grade SCC.

Melanocytic naevi

Degrees of pigmentation are common in melanocytic naevi, just as they are in BCC, but translucency is rarely a feature. In addition, intradermal naevi are, by definition, very long-standing. NMSC will be more recent in onset; this should be a clearly distinguishing feature.

Appendageal tumours

These grow from hair follicles and sweat glands and consequently present as nodules (Fig. 7.5). More than 20 varieties have been defined. Examples are apocrine hydrocystoma and trichoepithelioma, both of which are slow-growing, translucent, dome-shaped nodules usually located on the head and neck. They may be difficult to distinguish from BCC.

Table 7.1 Differential diagnosis of non-melanoma skin cancer

Types of pathology	Common examples
Premalignant and malignant	Actinic keratosis
	Keratoacanthoma
	Bowen's disease
	Other skin cancers
Hyperplasia	Sebaceous hyperplasia
	Pyogenic granuloma
Benign growths	Melanocytic naevi
	Appendageal tumours
	Cysts
	Seborrhoeic keratosis
	Chondrodermatitis
Infections	Molluscum
	Viral warts
	Tinea
	Folliculitis/acne
Others	Eczema, psoriasis
	Leg ulcers
	Granuloma annulare

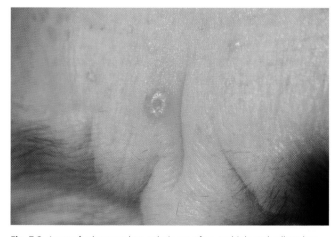

Fig. 7.3 Areas of sebaceous hyperplasia are often multiple and yellow, but otherwise share many features with small basal cell carcinoma.

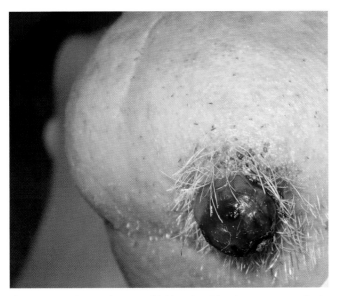

Fig. 7.4 Pyogenic granulomas are friable red nodules that grow over a short period of time (usually 2–6 weeks). They may resemble poorly differentiated skin tumours – compare this image with Fig. 7.12.

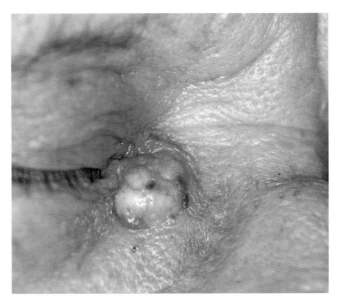

Fig. 7.6 Small epidermoid cysts are white and have a punctum, but may otherwise mimic basal cell carcinoma.

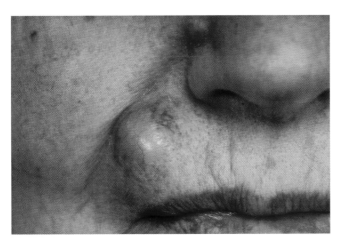

Fig. 7.5 Appendageal tumours vary from translucent cystic structures to red or mauve nodules.

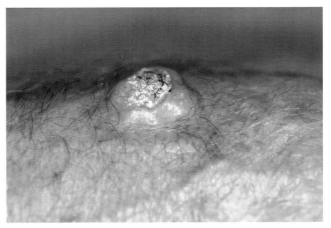

Fig. 7.7 Rapidly growing squamous cell carcinoma (SCC). This sort of lesion is occasionally confused with an infected or ruptured cyst. In SCC, the edge is non-tender, pink and hard, and there is no surrounding erythema. An inflamed cyst should be deformable and tender with evidence of a surrounding erythematous flare.

Cysts

Cysts tend to be white with a punctum, and are deformable if they contain soft keratin (Fig. 7.6). Similarly, milia are 1–2-mm, white firm superficial cysts which are normally easily diagnosable. An SCC may be misdiagnosed as an inflamed cyst, but these should be clinically distinguishable (Fig. 7.7). A useful sign in SCC is ulceration beneath the keratin plug.

Seborrhoeic keratosis

These great pretenders cause confusion with numerous clinical entities, including BCC. The stuck-on warty appearance and greasy, shiny or sometimes crumbly surface may help to tell them apart (Fig. 7.8).

Chondrodermatitis

Prominent areas of the helix or antehelix may develop a non-healing tender papule or ulcer. Compared with a BCC, chondrodermatitis is more likely to be erythematous, painful (particularly at night) and lacking the pearly edge and telangiectasias (Fig. 7.9).

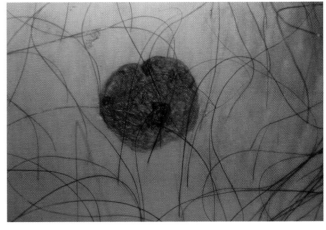

Fig. 7.8 Seborrhoeic keratosis. Here it has an unusual colour that can resemble basal cell carcinoma or poorly differentiated squamous cell carcinoma.

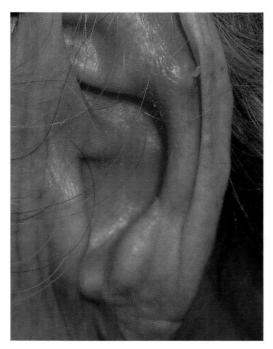

Fig. 7.9 Chondrodermatitis. There is a tender ulcerated nodule on the antehelix showing a characteristic scale overlying the lesion. Lesions develop on the prominent areas of the ear and may cause severe pain during the night.

Molluscum

Adults may have a solitary lesion that on the head or neck may be mistaken for a BCC (Fig. 7.10). With magnification the central keratin core is more obvious. Immunosuppression should be considered in adults who have large facial mollusca.

Scars

Morphoeic BCC resembling scar tissue may cause diagnostic problems, especially if recurrent, when it may be hard to differentiate from the original surgical scar.

Viral warts

Viral warts should present little difficulty with their well-organized structure and the typical stippled centre. In the elderly, differentiation from a hypertrophic AK or early SCC may not be so clear (Fig. 7.11). A useful clinical point is that viral warts do not bleed.

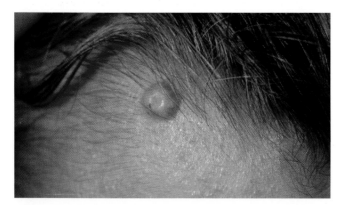

Fig. 7.10 Molluscum contagiosum is usually multiple in children. In adults, large solitary lesions are hard to distinguish from non-melanoma skin cancer.

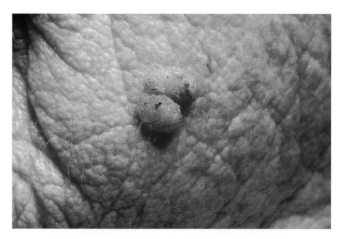

Fig. 7.11 Viral warts are less common in adults. Here the capillary thromboses, causing tiny black dots, are visible, but otherwise there are features in common with hyperkeratotic actinic keratosis or Bowen's disease and with squamous cell carcinoma.

Tinea

Ringworm may resemble a superficial BCC. However, in ringworm the centre clears and tiny pustules can appear at the periphery.

Inflamed spots due to folliculitis or acne

Inflammatory papules are often seen on the head, neck and hair-bearing skin. They tend to settle over a few days or weeks, but occasionally persist for months. Generally, an antibiotic cream helps these inflamed follicular lesions to heal, although they may take much longer to settle than anticipated.

Eczema and psoriasis

Small patches of these inflammatory disorders may be confused with superficial BCC. Psoriasis usually has a sharp margin, silvery scale and small bleeding points which appear on light scratching. BCC is fixed, whereas inflammatory skin lesions wax and wane.

Granuloma annulare

Small annular lesions with beaded papules on the hands may be confused with BCC.

Specific clinical situations

The red nodule

An unexplained, fast-growing red nodule should be treated with respect and needs urgent specialist assessment (Fig. 7.12). It may represent amelanotic melanoma (Fig. 8.9), aggressive variants of SCC (Fig. 5.4) or BCC, as well as rare skin cancers such as Merkel cell tumours, appendageal tumours, sarcoma, lymphoma and skin metastases. A friable, bleeding red nodule growing over 2–6 weeks may represent a pyogenic granuloma (Fig. 7.4).

Facial nodular lesions

A smooth papule or nodule with some translucence and possibly overlying telangiectasia is not uncommon on the face. Benign melanocytic naevi, appendageal tumours, sebaceous hyperplasia and small cysts all need to be considered in the differential diagnosis.

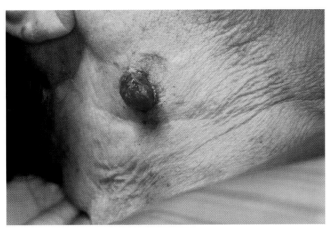

Fig. 7.12 Red nodules are potentially serious, as they can represent aggressive or poorly differentiated skin cancers as well as benign lesions such as pyogenic granulomas (compare this with Fig. 7.4). They therefore require urgent referral.

Cutaneous horns

Possible pathologies include viral wart, AK, Bowen's disease, seborrhoeic keratosis and SCC (Fig. 5.3). Overall there is a 15% chance that it will be malignant. Generally, a horn arising from normal flat epidermis is likely to be benign, whereas a fleshy base makes malignant change more likely. Also, a malignant horn tends to continue to grow.

Scaly lesions on the leg

Single or multiple red scaly patches on the lower limb are frequent in older people (Fig. 7.13). If a solitary patch of psoriasis or ringworm can be excluded, then Bowen's disease and superficial BCC must be considered. Even specialists have shown difficulty in distinguishing

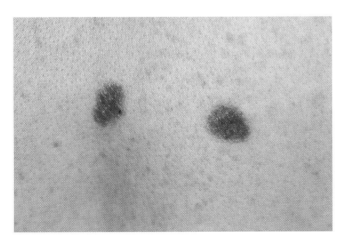

Fig. 7.13 This shows two superficial basal cell carcinomas (BCCs). Red patches, sometimes with a little scale, can be found on the trunk and limbs. If small areas of eczema and psoriasis can be ruled out, it remains difficult to distinguish between superficial BCC and Bowen's disease.

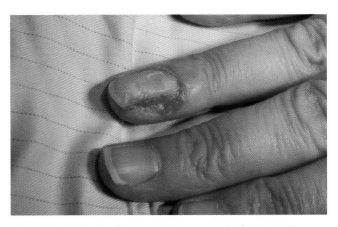

Fig. 7.14 This lesion had been treated as a paronychia for 2 years. Biopsy showed Bowen's disease with early transformation into squamous cell carcinoma.

these two pathologies when seen on the lower limb, missing the diagnosis of BCC in nearly 40% of cases.

Leg ulcers

A leg ulcer failing to respond to standard treatment will occasionally turn out to be malignant. This may be either SCC (a Marjolin's ulcer) or BCC (Fig. 5.6).

Radiation sites

Radiotherapy scars show progressive changes with time. There may be pallor, speckled pigmentation, prominent telangiectasia and breakdown of tissue into a necrotic ulcer (Fig. 12.7). This is often misinterpreted as recurrent skin cancer or development of a new cancer at the site of exposure to ionizing radiation, and a skin biopsy may be required.

Nail fold lesions

There may be delay in the diagnosis of skin cancers arising in the nail unit. This is usually due to inappropriate management of red, granulating, ulcerating, fixed, often non-tender lesions as paronychia. Paronychia is normally very tender; 'atypical paronychia' should be biopsied (Fig. 7.14).

Eyelid lesions

The eyelids may produce nodular BCC that resemble chalazion, infiltrative BCC appearing as a red lid and scarring BCC that present as subtle ectropion.

Further reading

Brown SJ, Lawrence CM. The management of skin malignancy: to what extent should we rely on clinical diagnosis? Br J Dermatol 2006; 155:100–3.
Colver GB. Skin cancer. A practical guide to management. Martin Dunitz, 2002
Harris AJ, Burge SM. Basal cell carcinomas on the legs: an under-diagnosed problem? Br J Dermatol 1996; 135 (Suppl. 47):22.

CHAPTER 8

Benign pigmented lesions

Sajjad Rajpar, Jerry Marsden

OVERVIEW

- It is essential to take a proper history and perform a thorough examination when assessing a pigmented lesion.
- Benign pigmented lesions are usually long-standing and have a history of little or no change in size, shape or colour.
- Acquired melanocytic naevi are the commonest pigmented lesions to be confused with melanoma in young adults. Most lesions start as junctional naevi, which progress over time to compound and then intradermal naevi.
- Atypical moles are a subset of acquired melanocytic naevi which are harder to distinguish from melanoma as they tend to be larger, more irregular and asymmetrical. The presence of many atypical moles increases the lifetime risk of melanoma.
- Seborrhoeic keratoses are the commonest pigmented lesions to be confused with melanoma in older adults. Most seborrhoeic keratoses appear as stuck-on lesions with a warty surface, although some are less typical and harder to diagnose on clinical grounds.
- There should be a low threshold for referral of pigmented lesions to a specialist if a confident diagnosis cannot be reached or if there is a possibility of melanoma.

The heightened public awareness of melanoma has led to increased numbers of patients requesting assessment of pigmented lesions. Most pigmented lesions presenting to general practitioners are benign and can be diagnosed on clinical grounds; a selection of the most common is discussed here.

Assessment of any pigmented lesion requires an accurate history to be taken and physical signs to be elicited (including inspection and palpation), and for the two to be integrated to reach a compatible diagnosis; spot diagnosis is dangerous and should always be avoided, however great the temptation. Benign pigmented lesions are normally long-standing and have a history of little or no change in size, shape or colour. Once a confident diagnosis is made, simple reassurance is usually sufficient. Treatment may be justified for the minority of lesions that are symptomatic. Referral to a dermatologist is necessary if a clinical diagnosis cannot be made, or if the history and physical signs are at odds with the proposed clinical diagnosis. For example, a history of rapid growth and bleeding is incompatible with a clinical diagnosis of a compound naevus. Similarly, in an adolescent, a new 5-mm dark brown macule would be consistent with a diagnosis of a junctional naevus. However, an identical lesion in a 60-year-old would be much more likely to be a solar lentigo or early melanoma. In general, a low threshold for referral of pigmented lesions is widely supported.

Freckles

Freckles occur on sun-exposed areas in individuals who have a tendency to sunburn easily, typically those with fair skin and red or blond hair. They normally appear before the age of 5 years as well-demarcated light brown macules with regular or irregular edges, up to 5 mm in diameter (Fig. 8.1). They fade in the winter, darken during the summer and disappear after the age of 20. Freckles have a normal number of epidermal melanocytes which produce more melanin than usual. They are not pre-cancerous, but occur in individuals with sun-sensitive skin who are in any case at greater risk of skin cancer.

Simple lentigo/solar lentigo

Lentigines are, like freckles, pigmented macules. However, unlike freckles, they contain an increased number of normal epidermal melanocytes. Simple lentigines are found in all races, and may be present at birth or develop at any age. They may be single, multiple or generalized and may occur anywhere, including the genitalia, mucus membranes and nail apparatus. Solar lentigines are simple lentigines that develop in the over 40s on sun-exposed skin.

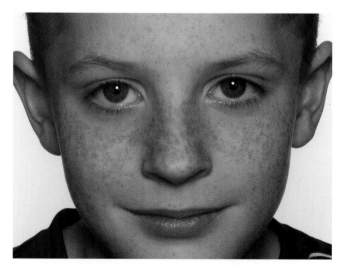

Fig. 8.1 Freckles. There are multiple pigmented macules on this boy's face.

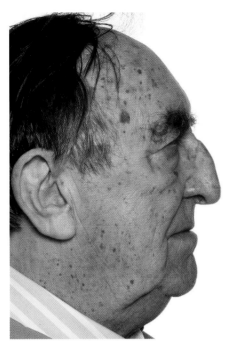

Fig. 8.2 Solar lentigines. There are multiple pigmented macules on the face of this man, who gave a history of excessive sun exposure. The raised pigmented lesions are seborrhoeic keratoses.

Lentigines are brown to black, well-demarcated macules usually 2–5 mm in diameter, although occasionally up to 10–15 mm (Fig. 8.2). They are darker than freckles and do not fluctuate in colour with sun exposure. It can be difficult to distinguish clinically between a simple lentigo and a junctional naevus or a flat pigmented seborrhoeic keratosis. The distinction from early superficial spreading melanoma is made on the history of a lesion that is changing and growing over a period of months and the presence of suggestive signs such as asymmetry and colour variegation. In an older individual, the diagnosis of lentigo maligna should be considered for an irregular facial lentigo (Fig. 4.9). If in doubt, excision for histological diagnosis may be required.

Café-au-lait macule

Café-au-lait macules are present at birth or develop during childhood, and like freckles contain a normal number of melanocytes that overproduce melanin. They are well-demarcated, brown macules measuring up to several centimetres, and are strikingly uniform in colour (Fig. 8.3). Single café-au-lait macules occur in 10–20% of White adults – more than six is unusual and suggestive of neurofibromatosis.

Congenital melanocytic naevus

Melanocytic naevi are present at birth or shortly after in 1% of individuals. Most are < 5 cm in diameter, and become darker, more palpable and verrucous during adolescence (Fig. 8.4). Risk of melanoma for lesions between 5 and 20 cm may be increased, but data on this are limited. It is reasonable to discuss the advantages and disadvantages of surgical excision with a specialist. Lesions that are > 20 cm ('giant' congenital melanocytic naevi) are rare and carry a definite increased risk of melanoma both in childhood and adulthood.

Acquired melanocytic naevus

Acquired melanocytic naevi (moles) develop between the ages of 5 and 30 years, particularly around puberty (Table 8.1). The number of melanocytic naevi peaks to an average of 20–30 in young adults aged 20–30 years. There is a progressive decline in number after this age, and no more than 5–10 lesions are usually present in the seventh decade. The number of melanocytic naevi directly predicts the risk of melanoma, so that individuals with > 100 lesions have a 7–11-fold greater risk of melanoma. It has been shown that sun protection in children reduces the development of melanocytic naevi.

It is likely that most acquired melanocytic naevi start as junctional naevi (Fig. 8.5), which progress over time to compound naevi (Fig. 8.6) and then intradermal naevi (Fig. 8.7). This means that in children and teenagers, most melanocytic naevi are junctional and compound, evolving to intradermal naevi in adults between 20 and 30 years. This is why a 'new junctional naevus' arising after the age of 35–40 years may well be an early melanoma. It is usual to have a mixture of different types of melanocytic naevi in an individual, although each lesion may not always go through every stage of evolution.

The vast majority of melanocytic naevi are completely harmless. The risk of malignant transformation is extremely low, and excising

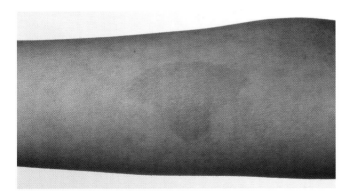

Fig. 8.3 Café-au-lait macule. There is a well-demarcated, uniformly coloured brown macule.

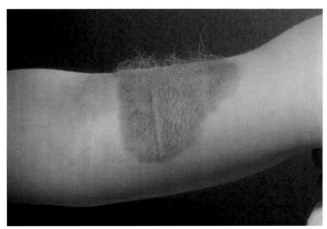

Fig. 8.4 Congenital melanocytic naevus. There is a fleshy papillomatous plaque with excessive growth of terminal hair.

Table 8.1 Clinical characteristics of junctional, compound and intradermal naevi

	Junctional naevus	Compound naevus	Intradermal naevus
Location of naevus cells	Dermo-epidermal junction	Dermo-epidermal junction and dermis	Dermis
History			
Age of appearance (years)	5–30	5–35	≥20
Change in size	Gradual increase in size as the child grows, and during pregnancy	Gradual increase in size as the child grows, and during pregnancy	Usually does not change in size
Examination			
Type of lesion	Macule	Papule with various degrees of elevation	Papule
Size (mm)	1–5	5–10	2–10
Colour	Light to dark brown – evenly coloured	Light to dark brown – evenly coloured	Brown, speckled, pink or skin coloured
Border	Well demarcated	Well demarcated	Well demarcated
Symmetry	Symmetrical	Symmetrical	Symmetrical
Differential diagnosis	Melanoma, simple lentigo, solar lentigo, freckle	Melanoma, seborrhoeic keratosis, dermatofibroma, haemangioma	Skin tag, basal cell carcinoma

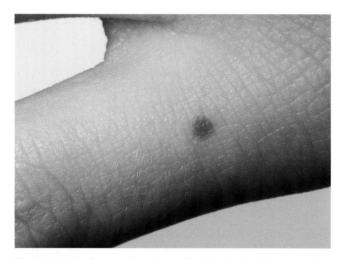

Fig. 8.5 Junctional naevus. There is a small and regular dark brown macule in an adolescent.

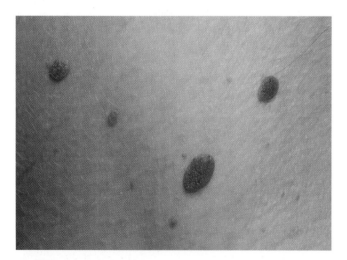

Fig. 8.6 Compound naevi. There are multiple, regular dark brown papules in a young adult. Lesions are soft and symmetrical.

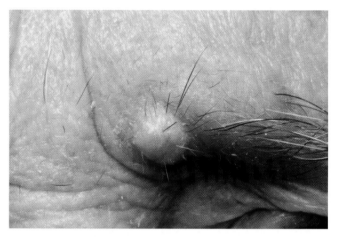

Fig. 8.7 Intradermal naevus. There is a soft, skin-coloured papule with hairs growing from it in this older adult.

them to prevent melanoma is not justified. Moreover, only 30–40% of melanomas develop in pre-existing melanocytic naevi, with the remainder arising on clinically normal skin. Occasionally, compound and intradermal naevi can become inflamed, indicated by a sudden development of redness, tenderness and swelling which settles over 4–6 weeks. Itching as the only feature of change in a melanocytic naevus is not predictive of melanoma, although it is often a major concern among patients.

Halo naevus

Occasionally, an immunological reaction to naevus cells leads to a halo of vitiligo-like depigmentation around a melanocytic naevus, followed by disappearance of the lesion altogether (Fig. 8.8). Such 'halo naevi' do not need specific treatment as long as the melanocytic naevus appears benign. Repigmentation may take several months and does not always occur.

Atypical mole (dysplastic naevus)

This is a controversial term that is difficult to define consistently. It encompasses acquired melanocytic naevi that may be larger, have irregular or ill-defined borders, or have irregular pigmentation compared with ordinary acquired naevi (Fig. 8.9). The borders may blur into the surrounding skin, and there may be redness that blanches

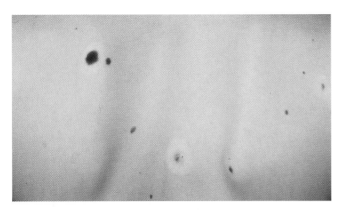

Fig. 8.8 Halo naevi. There is a vitiliginous rim of depigmentation around several benign melanocytic naevi in this adolescent. The patient should be reassured.

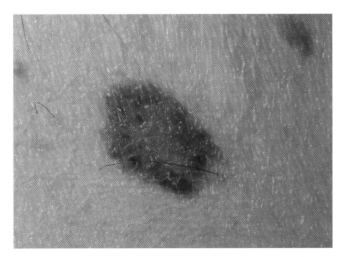

Fig. 8.9 Atypical mole. Atypical moles can be difficult to discriminate from melanoma.

with the pressure of a glass slide. These features are less than expected in early melanoma, and a history that the lesion has recently changed or expanded in size is usually absent. Even so, distinction from early melanoma with confidence may be difficult, and referral for specialist assessment is often required. Excision of an atypical mole is necessary only if an experienced clinician is uncertain about the diagnosis. Histological analysis reveals dysplasia, without the features of melanoma. Atypical moles are quite common and may occur in up to 5–10% of individuals. The presence of large numbers of moles and moles which are atypical is known as the Atypical Mole syndrome (Box 1.1; Fig. 1.2) and is a powerful independent risk factor for melanoma. This occurs in up to 2% of the population. Again, most melanoma in patients with atypical moles do not occur in pre-existing lesions. It is therefore not justified to excise atypical moles for melanoma prevention.

Seborrhoeic keratosis

Seborrhoeic keratoses (basal cell papilloma, senile warts) account for 25–30% of referrals for melanoma screening. Consequently, it is important to understand their natural history and range of appearance. Seborrhoeic keratoses are common benign epidermal tumours

derived from keratinocytes. Prevalence studies from the UK show that they are present in 30% of those aged 40–50 years, and 70% of those >70 years. The number and size of lesions increase with age, and an average adult has anywhere between 10 and 60 lesions. There is a relationship to sun exposure – the prevalence is higher in Australia, where lesions are present in 16% of teenagers aged 15–19 years.

Seborrhoeic keratoses are usually ovoid and may be skin coloured, pink, light brown, dark brown, grey or black (Fig. 8.10). Approximately two-thirds are pigmented, two-thirds are flat and two-thirds measure >3 mm in diameter (up to 2 or 3 cm in some cases). They usually have a stuck-on appearance, and look as if they can be easily 'peeled' off. The surface is typically soft and crumbly. Flat lesions have a dull matt surface and characteristically increased skin lines. Lesions may become irritated and inflamed, sometimes for several weeks, but will settle with topical antiseptics and dressings.

Seborrhoeic keratoses are usually easy to diagnose, but may occasionally present as shiny, darkly pigmented papules (Fig. 8.11) or flat darkly pigmented featureless macules. These can be very difficult to

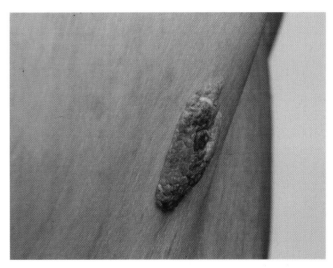

Fig. 8.10 Seborrhoeic keratosis. This typical lesion has a stuck-on appearance and a 'crumbly', warty surface.

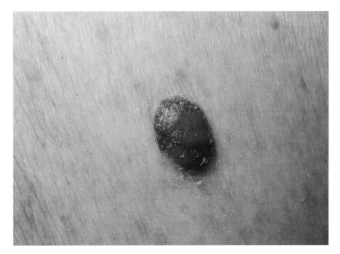

Fig. 8.11 Seborrhoeic keratosis. This lesion is a darkly and irregularly pigmented shiny nodule and is difficult to distinguish from nodular melanoma.

distinguish from melanoma without careful assessment. This may include dermatoscopy, which should show the characteristic keratin plugging and keratin cysts. Seborrhoeic keratoses are not premalignant and do not need treatment unless symptomatic.

Dermatofibroma

Dermatofibroma (benign fibrous histiocytoma) is a benign tumour that consists of fibroblasts and histiocytes. It most commonly appears on the lower legs of women as a firm dermal papule or nodule measuring 5–10 mm in diameter (Fig. 8.12). The overlying skin is grey, brown or pink. Palpation is particularly helpful in diagnosis, as thickening of the skin is felt beyond the visible boundaries, and pinching the lesion causes dimpling in the centre since they are confined to the dermis. This sign is suggestive but not diagnostic of dermatofibroma. Lesions usually grow slowly, then become static in size and persist for many years. Most lesions are asymptomatic, although some may be itchy.

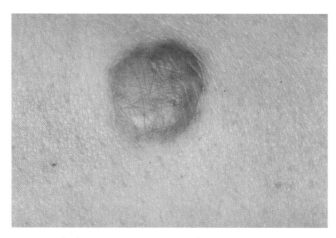

Fig. 8.12 Dermatofibroma. There is a firm, light brown nodule.

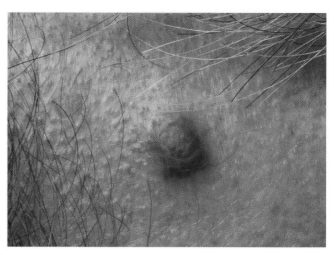

Fig. 8.13 Haemangioma. There is a purple compressible papule. Individual dilated vascular channels can be seen.

Haemangiomas

Acquired haemangiomas are common and consist of dilated dermal blood vessels. They are 2–5-mm, red or purple papules which may blanch on pressure (Fig. 8.13). Occasionally, they may be very dark and difficult to distinguish from nodular melanoma.

Further reading

Krengel S, Hauschild A, Schafer T. Melanoma risk in congenital melanocytic naevi: a systematic review. Br J Dermatol 2006; 155:1–8.

Matz H, Orion E, Ruocco V, Wolf R. Clinical simulators of melanoma. Clin Dermatol 2002; 20:212–21.

Memon AA, Tomenson JA, Bothwell J, Friedmann PS. Prevalence of solar damage and actinic keratoses in a Merseyside population. Br J Dermatol 2000; 142:1154-9.

Naeyaert JM, Brochez L. Clinical practice. Dysplastic naevi. N Engl J Med 2003; 349:2233–40.

CHAPTER 9

Melanoma – clinical features and diagnosis

Sajjad Rajpar, Jerry Marsden

OVERVIEW

- The commonest locations for melanoma are the legs of women and the trunk of men.

- Most melanomas have a history of being new or of having changed in size, shape or colour.

- The ABCDE criteria are an easy aide memoir for screening pigmented lesions. They are useful for detecting superficial spreading melanoma, but less useful for nodular melanoma, amelanotic melanoma and early melanoma.

- It is appropriate to refer a new or changing pigmented lesion for a specialist opinion unless it is certain that the lesion is benign. Similarly, a lesion that has features suspicious of melanoma, but where a history of change is lacking, should also be referred.

- 2% of melanomas are amelanotic and do not produce any pigment.

- Serial photography and dermatoscopy are increasingly used in dermatological practice to help detect early melanoma. Other non-invasive methods of diagnosis are an active area of investigation.

It is only possible to diagnose melanoma definitively once a lesion has been excised and analysed histologically. However, the preceding step, which is to clinically identify lesions that are suspicious enough to require excision, is central to the management of melanoma, with the goal being to identify lesions at an early stage when they are thin and complete excision is curative. Several studies have shown that the accuracy of clinical diagnosis of melanoma improves with level of clinical experience. Even so, an average of four to five benign lesions are excised for every melanoma in dedicated pigmented lesion screening clinics, highlighting the difficulty in clinically differentiating melanoma from benign lesions, even among experts. This is explained by the wide variation in the clinical morphology of melanoma, which overlaps with the wide variation in morphology of benign lesions (Fig. 9.1). The variations in the appearance of melanoma can be attributed to:

- Clinical subtype
- Progression (how advanced a lesion is)
- Degree of pigmentation.

The best way to avoid missing a melanoma is to take an accurate history, examine the lesion carefully and critically fit this together to make a diagnosis that is consistent with the observations. The main clinical features that help distinguish melanoma from benign lesions can be remembered easily as an acronym: ABCDE (Table 9.1). 'Spot' diagnosis is dangerous and should be avoided. Tools such as dermatoscopy, which may aid the *in vivo* diagnosis of melanoma, are increasingly used in clinical practice.

ABCDE criteria

The first four criteria are static features that can be appreciated on examination, whereas the final criterion of 'evolution' assesses the dynamicity of the lesion and is ascertained from the history. There is a 99.8% chance that lesions lacking any of the ABCDE criteria are not melanoma, but only a 1.5% probability of melanoma if any single criterion is met (assuming a population prevalence of 1%). Hence, each criterion is sensitive but not specific for the diagnosis of melanoma, with specificity improving significantly when more than one criterion are present. Practically, the presence of one feature should raise alertness, and two or more features should prompt urgent referral for a specialist opinion. However, if there are strong concerns, any one feature is adequate to prompt urgent referral.

History
Key questions in the history are whether the lesion is new, and whether it is changing in size, shape or colour, as the premise of the 'evolu-

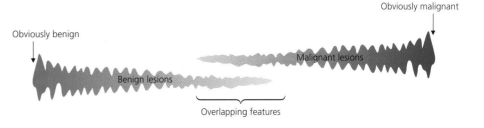

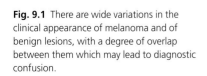

Fig. 9.1 There are wide variations in the clinical appearance of melanoma and of benign lesions, with a degree of overlap between them which may lead to diagnostic confusion.

Table 9.1 Modified American Cancer Society's ABCDE criteria

	Benign naevus	SSM	Nodular melanoma
Asymmetry – one half of the lesion not identical to the other, either in shape or colour	No	Yes	Not always
Border irregularity – lesion has an uneven or ragged border	No	Yes	Not always
Colour variegation – lesion has more than one colour (i.e. black, blue, grey, red, white or skin colour)	No	Yes	Sometimes
Diameter – lesion has a diameter >6 mm	Occasionally	Yes	Yes
Evolving – new lesion or history of change in size, shape or colour	Sometimes	Always	Always

This scheme is more useful for detecting SSM than nodular melanoma, amelanotic melanoma or early melanoma.
SSM, Superficial spreading melanoma.

tion' criterion is that melanoma grows and changes. Two-thirds of melanoma are new lesions, with the remainder developing from pre-existing benign melanocytic naevi. As it is unusual to develop new benign naevi after the age of 30 years, new pigmented lesions developing after this age should be scrutinized carefully for melanoma. Melanoma typically darkens, increases in size and becomes more irregular in outline over a period of 2–12 months. Change in colour tends to be noticed by patients before a change in size or shape. It is appropriate to refer a new or changing pigmented lesion for a specialist opinion unless it is certain that the lesion is benign and that the degree of change is 'normal' for that lesion.

Change in a pigmented lesion over a couple of weeks is almost invariably due to inflammation or trauma, as in an inflamed seborrhoeic keratosis. Bleeding and pain are features of very advanced melanomas, but also occur with irritated or excoriated benign lesions. The presence of itch does not help discriminate between melanoma and other lesions. In some cases a history is unavailable, such as for lesions on the back, and reliance must be placed on the clinical examination.

Examination

The commonest locations for melanoma are the legs of women and the trunk of men, although any site may be affected (Fig. 9.2). The static elements of the ABCDE criteria fit best with superficial spreading melanoma (SSM). Caution must be exercised when applying these criteria to nodular, amelanotic or early melanomas, as asymmetry and irregularity in colour may not necessarily be present. In an individual with many naevi, one that stands out deserves closer inspection. With experience, the ABCDE features are often assimilated into an intuitive impression of the overall architecture of a lesion.

Clinical subtypes

There are four subtypes of melanoma, each with characteristic clinical and histological appearances (Table 9.2). The subtype does not influ-

ence prognosis, which is related, in all instances, to the vertical tumour thickness measured histologically – known as the Breslow thickness (Fig. 10.2).

Superficial spreading melanoma

SSM is the commonest subtype and is most frequently found on the legs of women and the trunk of men (Fig. 9.3 and Fig. 9.9). Lesions grow outwards over months to years (radial growth), accumulating foci of various colours, including brown, black, grey and red, as they mature. They subsequently become nodular in areas, indicating the lesion has entered vertical growth. The period of radial growth gives an opportunity to detect these melanomas when they are relatively thin.

Nodular melanoma

Nodular melanoma typically presents as a rapidly expanding dark brown or black nodule that ulcerates and bleeds (Fig. 9.4). Lesions are most commonly found on the trunk, although any body site can be affected, including covered areas such as the axillae and buttocks. Recognition may be delayed because an irregular edge and multiple colours are often absent. As growth is rapid and vertical from the outset, they are often thicker than SSM at diagnosis and consequently associated with a higher mortality.

Lentigo maligna melanoma

Lentigo maligna (LM) is a specific type of melanoma *in situ* that de-

Table 9.2 Clinical subtypes of melanoma, relative frequency and typical age range at diagnosis

Clinical subtype	Relative frequency (%)	Age range at diagnosis (years)
Superficial spreading melanoma	75	30–60
Nodular melanoma	15	40–80
Lentigo maligna melanoma	5–10	>60
Acral melanoma	<5	–

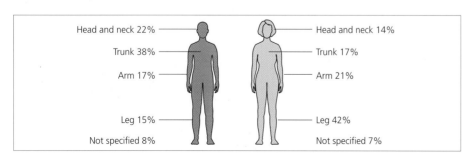

Head and neck 22% Head and neck 14%
Trunk 38% Trunk 17%
Arm 17% Arm 21%
Leg 15% Leg 42%
Not specified 8% Not specified 7%

Fig. 9.2 Percentage distribution of melanoma on parts of the body.

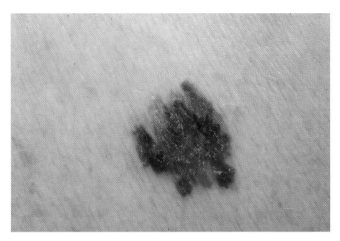

Fig. 9.3 Superficial spreading melanoma. There is an asymmetric lesion, with irregular borders and multiple shades of brown, grey, pink and black.

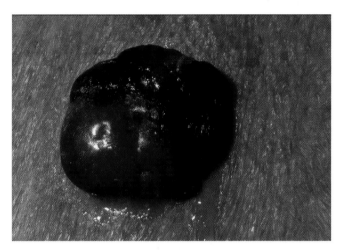

Fig. 9.4 Nodular melanoma. There is an ulcerated and haemorrhagic black nodule. The prognosis of this sort of melanoma is poor.

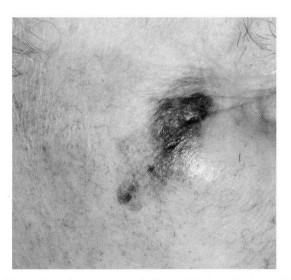

Fig. 9.5 Lentigo maligna melanoma. A thickened black area (melanoma) has developed in the medial portion of a long-standing irregular brown macule (lentigo maligna).

velops in chronically sun-exposed areas, particularly the face, in the elderly (Fig. 4.9). Because it is *in situ*, i.e. confined to the epidermis, LM is impalpable. It grows radially, often over several years, as an irregular tan to dark-brown macule. Over time, 5–15% of LM lesions develop areas of invasive melanoma (Fig. 9.5). Areas that have transformed into LM melanoma darken and become palpable, as a papule, nodule or plaque. These are usually late signs of invasive transformation. Early invasion is difficult to detect clinically, and 5–10% of lesions thought to be LM clinically are shown to have foci of invasive disease when they are analysed after excision.

Acral and nail melanoma

Acral and nail melanomas are rare. They are not thought to be caused by excessive sun exposure, and are the commonest melanoma subtype in racially pigmented populations. Acral melanoma occurs more frequently on the soles than on the palms. Lesions appear as brown or grey pigmented macules with or without papules or ulceration (Fig. 9.6). These abnormalities may be masked by reactive hyperkeratosis, and lesions may consequently look verrucous or scaly. It is important to consider this diagnosis in solitary non-healing foot lesions, particularly if ulcerated. Nail melanoma affects the great toe more than any other digit, usually starting under the cuticle and producing a pigmented streak in the nail plate.

Progression

Advanced lesions are generally easier to identify clinically as melanoma, as a number of the ABCDE features are often apparent. Early melanoma is more subtle and requires a lower index of suspicion. Very early lesions typically have a history of change, with some element of irregularity of the borders and colour variation. They tend to be small, often < 6 mm in diameter. In some series, almost one in five excised melanomas are melanoma *in situ* (excluding LM), where the malignant cells are confined to the epidermis. If left alone, it is believed that *in situ* lesions progress to invasive melanoma.

Degree of pigmentation

Two per cent of melanoma produces very little or no pigment (Fig. 9.7).

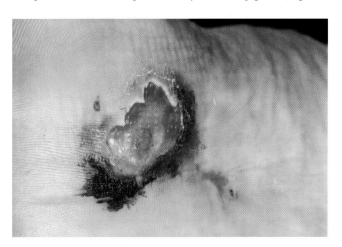

Fig. 9.6 Acral melanoma. There is an ulcer on the sole of the foot, with irregular pigmented borders.

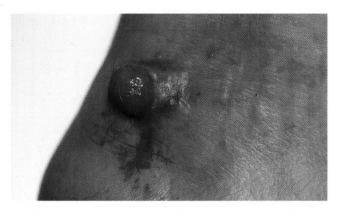

Fig. 9.7 Amelanotic nodular melanoma. There is an eroded haemorrhagic nodule that is devoid of any pigment.

Lesions are pink to red in colour and may be mistaken for basal cell carcinoma or benign growths.

Tools to aid *in vivo* diagnosis of melanoma

Several methods of lesion analysis that may improve clinical accuracy are being investigated, although photography and dermatoscopy are the only ones in current clinical practice (Fig. 9.8).

Individual lesion photography

Baseline photography is frequently performed for individual pigmented lesions that have a very low likelihood of being malignant and so do not warrant excision. Patients are seen at a fixed interval so that comparison with baseline photographs can be made and lack of progression confirmed. This approach is specifically restricted to patients whose lesions have been diagnosed as probably benign, but in whom there is a small degree of uncertainty.

Total body cutaneous photography

The complete skin is photographed, and patients are clinically examined or re-photographed at regular intervals so that comparison can be made with baseline photographs for any new or changing lesions, which are then scrutinized more carefully. This sort of surveillance has been reported to increase early detection of melanoma in individuals at high risk who have large numbers

of melanocytic naevi. However, it is expensive, labour intensive and has not been compared with surveillance by clinicians or patients.

Dermatoscopy

Dermatoscopy (syn. dermoscopy) is becoming increasingly popular among dermatologists, as it adds complementary information to the clinical examination and can be performed with relative ease in the outpatient setting with a hand-held device. A liquid interface between the lens and the skin (alcohol gel or mineral oil) allows visualization immediately beneath the surface of the skin with

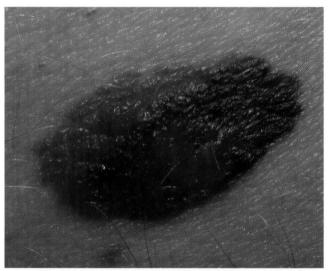

(a)

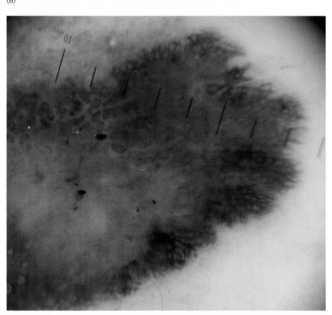

(b)

Fig. 9.9 (a) Clinical and (b) dermatoscopic image of a superficial spreading melanoma. There are several melanoma-specific features, including asymmetry, atypical pigment network, blue-grey veil and regression that become apparent on dermatoscopic examination. (Courtesy of Dr Sid Orpin, Solihull Hospital.)

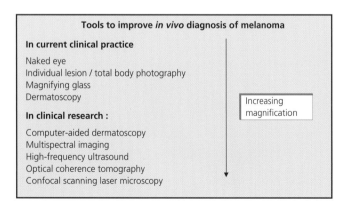

Tools to improve *in vivo* diagnosis of melanoma
In current clinical practice
Naked eye
Individual lesion / total body photography
Magnifying glass
Dermatoscopy
In clinical research :
Computer-aided dermatoscopy
Multispectral imaging
High-frequency ultrasound
Optical coherence tomography
Confocal scanning laser microscopy

Increasing magnification

Fig. 9.8 Tools to improve *in vivo* diagnosis of melanoma in current clinical practice and in clinical research.

10-fold magnification. Several morphological features become apparent, including pigment architecture and blood vessel arrangement (Fig. 9.9).

Dermatoscopy is particularly useful at identifying certain benign lesions such as seborrhoeic keratosis and haemangioma, which have specific dermatoscopic features. Differentiating benign melanocytic naevi from melanoma is harder, and requires considerable training and experience.

Tools in clinical research

Several other imaging modalities that offer higher magnifications at higher resolutions are being investigated. At this stage, no system has yet received adequate validation through rigorous clinical investigation, although it is likely that non-invasive screening technologies such as these will gain increasing recognition in the future.

Further reading

Abbasi NR, Shaw HM, Rigel DS *et al.* Early diagnosis of cutaneous melanoma: revisiting the ABCD criteria. JAMA 2004; 292:2771–6.

Braun RP, Rabinovitz HS, Oliviero M *et al.* Dermoscopy of pigmented skin lesions. J Am Acad Dermatol 2005; 52:109–21.

MacKie RM. Malignant melanoma: clinical variants and prognostic indicators. Clin Exp Dermatol 2000; 25:471–5.

Marghoob AA, Swindle LD, Moricz CZ *et al.* Instruments and new technologies for the *in vivo* diagnosis of melanoma. J Am Acad Dermatol 2003; 49:777–97.

Strayer SM, Reynolds PM. Diagnosing skin malignancy: assessment of predictive clinical criteria and risk factors. J Fam Pract 2003; 52:210–8.

CHAPTER 10

Melanoma – management and prognosis

Sajjad Rajpar, Jerry Marsden

OVERVIEW

- In the UK, patients with suspected melanoma should be referred for further assessment and management to a skin cancer multi-disciplinary team.
- Wider excision is the only curative treatment for melanoma. The size of wider excision margins is based on the Breslow thickness.
- The overall 5-year survival rate for melanoma is 80% for men and 90% for women.
- Breslow thickness and ulceration are the most important predictors of survival in clinical practice.
- Sentinel lymph node biopsy is a powerful predictor of survival, but has no established therapeutic benefit.
- There are currently no effective adjuvant therapies for melanoma.
- Eighty per cent of metastases develop within 5 years of diagnosis. The first site of metastasis is loco-regional in two-thirds of patients and distant in the remaining third.
- Melanoma is relatively resistant to conventional chemotherapy. Immunotherapy and targeted molecular therapy may lead to improved therapeutic responses in the future.

In the UK, patients with suspected melanoma are referred for assessment and management to a skin cancer multidisciplinary team (Table 10.1). Wider excision is usually curative in patients with thin melanoma (Breslow thickness <1 mm). Since most melanoma is thin, the overall 5-year survival rates are 90% for women and 80% for men in the UK. Thicker melanoma is more likely to metasta-

Table 10.1 Members of a skin cancer multidisciplinary team are from different backgrounds and have the skills and expertise required for the comprehensive management of skin cancers

Key members	Extended team members
Dermatologists	Palliative care specialists
Surgeons	Counsellors
Dermatopathologists	Psychologists
Primary care accredited practitioners	Cosmetic camouflage advisers
Skin cancer clinical nurse specialist	Prosthetists
Oncologists	Physiotherapist
Radiologists	Lympho-oedema specialist
Departmental nurses	Pharmacist

size. Metastatic melanoma responds poorly to chemotherapy and radiotherapy, although surgical treatment of local and lymph node metastases may still be curative. Immuno- and molecular therapy are being actively investigated.

Management

Primary (diagnostic) excision

A lesion suspected of being melanoma must be excised completely for histopathological analysis (Fig. 10.1). Punch or shave biopsies should be avoided because of possible sampling error and distortion of histological architecture compromising pathological diagnosis. A specialist dermatopathologist must report suspected melanoma, and correlation between clinical and histological findings is essential if misdiagnosis is to be avoided. Melanoma diagnosis must include measurement of the Breslow thickness (Fig. 10.2). This is the distance from the granular layer of the epidermis to the lower most invasive cell. This measurement predicts the risk of metastasis, and therefore survival.

Wider excision

Definitive treatment of melanoma involves excision of a safety margin of normal surrounding skin to the deep muscle fascia (Figs 8.8

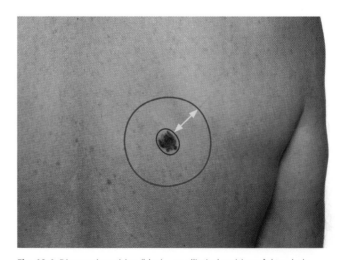

Fig. 10.1 Diagnostic excision (blue) – an elliptical excision of the whole lesion with narrow margins of 1–2 mm is performed. Wider excision (red) – definitive treatment comprises full-thickness excision of a 1–3-cm margin of skin (yellow) depending on the Breslow thickness of the primary melanoma.

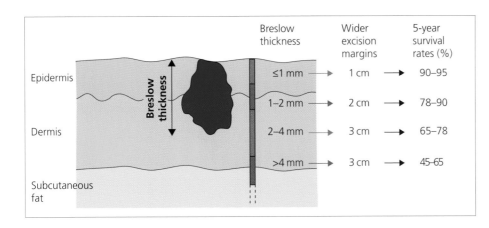

Fig. 10.2 The Breslow thickness is the distance from the granular layer of the epidermis to the deepest point of the tumour. It predicts the risk of metastasis, and therefore the 5-year survival rate of melanoma. The Breslow thickness determines the size of margins required for wider excision.

and 10.1). This is central to the successful management of melanoma, because it minimizes the risk of local and regional lymph node metastasis. The size of the wider margin is determined by the Breslow thickness. A margin of 1 cm is generally accepted for melanoma with a thickness of ≤ 1 mm. For melanoma between 1 and 2 mm in thickness, margins of 2 cm are probably adequate. Melanoma thicker than 2 mm requires margins of 3 cm. Most wider excision surgery takes place under local anaesthetic in the ambulatory care setting.

Staging and prognosis

Survival from primary melanoma is determined by Breslow thickness and the presence or absence of ulceration. These characteristics are used to define the American Joint Committee on Cancer staging system (Table 10.2; Fig. 10.3).

Table 10.2 Simplified version of the American Joint Committee on Cancer (AJCC) staging system for cutaneous melanoma. (Adapted from Balch CM et al. J Clin Oncol 2001; 19:3635–48.) Prognosis for primary melanoma is based on the Breslow thickness and presence or absence of ulceration

Stage		5-year survival rate (%)
I	≤1.0 mm without ulceration	95
	≤1.0 mm with ulceration	91
	1.01–2.0 mm without ulceration	89
II	1.01–2.0 mm with ulceration	77
	2.01–4.0 mm without ulceration	79
	2.01–4.0 mm with ulceration, or	63
	>4.0 mm without ulceration	67
	>4.0 mm with ulceration	45
III	Non-ulcerated primary of any depth and:	
	1 metastatic regional lymph node	59
	2–3 metastatic regional lymph nodes	46
	≥4 metastatic regional lymph nodes	27
	Ulcerated primary of any depth and	
	1 metastatic regional lymph node	29
	2–3 metastatic regional lymph nodes	25
	≥4 metastatic regional lymph nodes	13
IV	Metastasis to distant skin, distant lymph nodes, solid organs or bone	7–19

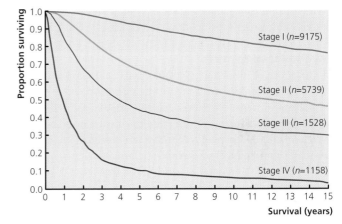

Fig. 10.3 Kaplan–Meier survival curves showing the relationship between stage and survival. From Balch CM et al. J Clin Oncol 2001; 19:3635–48 (with permission).

Sentinel lymph node biopsy

Sentinel lymph node biopsy (SNLB) adds accurate staging information for patients with primary melanoma. Radioactive tracer and blue dye are used to define the first lymph node draining the primary melanoma – the sentinel node. If melanoma is present in the sentinel lymph node, the 5-year survival averages at 50–60% compared with 90% if the sentinel lymph node is clear. Although SNLB provides patients with a better idea of their prognosis, there is no proven therapeutic value from early lymph node block dissection if a sentinel lymph node is positive. In the UK, SNLB is regarded as a clinical trial procedure.

Adjuvant treatment

Adjuvant treatment should eradicate micrometastases before they cause disease. Unfortunately, there are currently no effective adjuvant therapies for melanoma. Interferon-alfa, a proinflammatory cytokine, is the only licensed adjuvant treatment for melanoma, but its effect is limited to delaying metastases in some patients. Extensive investigation has shown only a 1–3% improvement in survival and is associated with significant toxicity and cost. Several other adjuvant therapies have been investigated, including interleukin-2, tamoxifen and melanoma-specific vaccines, although none has provided consistent benefit.

Breaking the news

The outlook varies enormously between patients, depending on tumour thickness and ulceration. It is therefore important to individualize prognosis when breaking bad news and to remain realistic while providing hope, reassurance and support. For example, *in situ* melanoma (where malignant melanocytes are confined to the epidermis) does not carry a risk of metastasis and so the patient would be strongly reassured. On the other hand, a 4-mm thick ulcerated melanoma carries a 5-year survival rate of 45%. In practice, once the word 'cancer' has been used, patients take in little further information. Consequently, a specialist nurse is a vital contact for further support, advice and counselling, and should be involved as early on in the process as possible, preferably from the time the bad news is broken.

Psychosocial aspects

The diagnosis of melanoma can have significant psychosocial impact, particularly because there is a widespread awareness among the public that it may be lethal. Feelings include vulnerability, fear, depression, anxiety and panic. Psychosocial distress impairs ability to cope, quality of life and possibly even survival. Providing general information on coping strategies and cognitive behavioural therapy (such as relaxation training) to patients with high levels of psychosocial distress improves quality of life and general health status of melanoma patients, underpinning the need for psychological support following diagnosis.

Metastatic melanoma

Eighty per cent of metastases develop within 5 years of diagnosis. Delayed recurrences, even decades after diagnosis, are well documented. The first site of metastasis is loco-regional in 60–80% of patients (Table 10.3). Surgical excision is the mainstay of treatment for metastatic disease, as systemic chemotherapy and immunotherapy have little effect. Radiotherapy has some role in the palliation of bone and cerebral metastases.

Loco-regional metastases

Satellite and in-transit metastases present as papules and nodules in the skin and subcutaneous tissues between the site of the original melanoma and the regional lymph nodes. They are treated by surgical

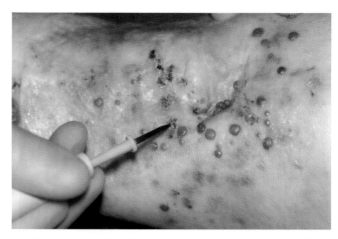

Fig. 10.4 Hyfrecation of multiple in-transit melanoma metastases on a limb. Symptomatic treatment is necessary as lesions may be painful or bleed. The hyfrecator emits a high-frequency current producing a spark at the tip of the electrode, which burns tissue superficially.

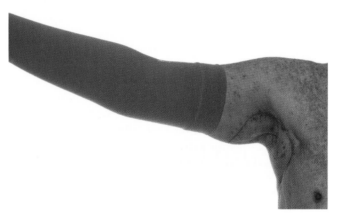

Fig. 10.5 This patient has had a right axillary lymph node block dissection for metastatic melanoma. Lympho-oedema is a common post-operative complication and requires compression hosiery.

excision, hyfrecation or carbon dioxide laser ablation or regional chemotherapy (Fig. 10.4). Metastasis to the regional lymph nodes presents with palpable lymphadenopathy and is treated by lymph node block dissection (Fig. 10.5). The prognosis from regional lymph node metastasis depends on the number of lymph nodes involved. For example, a patient with a non-ulcerated primary melanoma and a single metastatic lymph node has almost a 60% chance of cure. This means loco-regional metastases should be actively and aggressively treated.

Distant metastases

The prognosis for patients with distant metastasis is poor. The median survival is 6 months for visceral metastasis and 9–12 months for distant skin metastasis. Surgical excision of distant metastases is central to effective palliative care, and improves survival for isolated pulmonary, cerebral or gastrointestinal metastases (Fig. 10.6). Melanoma is relatively resistant to conventional chemotherapy with dacarbazine, which has been used for > 30 years and yields, at best, only a 15% response rate. Many of these responses are not clinically

Table 10.3 First site of metastasis in melanoma

Loco-regional – stage III (60–80%)	Distant – stage IV (20–40%)
• Regional lymph nodes • Satellite metastases (skin or subcutaneous tissues immediately around the original melanoma) • In-transit metastases (skin or subcutaneous tissues between original melanoma and regional lymph node)	• Solid organs • Skeleton • Distant skin • Distant lymph nodes

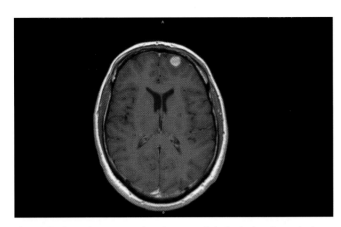

Fig. 10.6 Magnetic resonance imaging scan of the brain showing a single melanoma metastasis on the right frontal lobe. As there was no disease elsewhere, this lesion was treated by surgical excision.

Box 10.1 **Objectives for follow-up consultations**

- Detailed history for symptoms suggestive of melanoma metastases. These may be non-specific (fatigue) or specific (haemoptysis, headache, oedema)
- Examine original site for satellite and in-transit recurrence
- Examine for regional lymphadenopathy, distant lymphadenopathy and hepatomegaly
- Complete skin examination for further primary skin malignancies and premalignant lesions
- Reinforce photoprotection
- Promote self-examination (see Fig. 3.8), which should be:
  - demonstrated to all patients
  - supplemented with an information leaflet
  - performed every 2 months
  - comprehensive and include examination of primary site for recurrence, regional and distant lymph nodes for metastases, and complete skin for further skin malignancies.
- Identify patients with moderate to high psychosocial distress and offer appropriate psychological interventions.

relevant and there is no survival benefit. Patients should have access to palliative care teams for symptomatic control of advanced disease.

Follow-up

Follow-up for patients with melanoma enables earlier detection of metastatic disease and of new skin cancers, so that prompt, potentially curative, surgical intervention can be provided (Box 10.1). Follow-up also provides the opportunity to offer education and psychological support and to reinforce self-examination techniques, as up to 5% of patients develop a second primary melanoma, representing a 5–10-fold increased risk compared with the general population. Current UK guidelines suggest 3-monthly follow-up for 3 years for all newly diagnosed patients, followed by 6-monthly follow-up for a further 2 years for patients with melanoma thickness > 1 mm. Stage III and IV patients usually have follow-up at 3–6-monthly intervals for 10 years. In some areas, follow-up is shared by primary and secondary care services. Investigations at follow-up visits are usually guided by the history and physical examination.

Future directions

New chemotherapy agents introduced over the last 30 years have not shown any benefit over dacarbazine, even in multiple combinations, underlining the highly chemoresistant nature of melanoma. The complex molecular basis for this is becoming more apparent, and several new molecular targets have been identified with targeted agents undergoing pre-clinical and early clinical studies (Table 10.4).

The observation that melanoma can, on rare occasions, spontaneously regress has led to significant interest in immunotherapy,

Table 10.4 New therapeutic strategies for melanoma

	Problem	Solution
Chemotherapy	Resistant to chemotherapy-induced apoptosis	• Combine with immunotherapy and molecular therapy • Await new chemotherapy agents
Immunotherapy	• Tolerance to melanoma antigens making traditional vaccines less effective	• Dendritic cell vaccines • Heat shock protein-based vaccines • Concurrent use of proinflammatory agents such as interleukin-2
	• Different melanoma antigens between and within patients	• Polyvalent vaccines
Molecular therapy	Anti-apoptotic mechanisms in melanoma include • Over expression of Bcl-2 • Inactivation of APAF-1 by methylation • Overexpression of BRAF	Targeted therapy : • Antisense Bcl-2 oligonucleotides • Demethylating agents • BRAF inhibitors

APAF-1: Apoptosis protease activating factor-1.

including vaccines against melanoma antigens. So far, vaccines have produced low response rates and have not improved survival. The occasional striking improvement continues to fuel interest.

Clinical trials

The inefficacy of systemic therapies for melanoma makes it important for patients at high risk of metastasis and those with advanced melanoma to be enrolled into well-designed multicentre clinical trials. In the UK, information on ongoing clinical melanoma trials can be obtained from the National Cancer Research Institute.

Further reading

Balch CM, Buzaid AC, Soong SJ *et al*. Final version of the American Joint Committee on Cancer staging system for cutaneous melanoma. J Clin Oncol 2001; 19:3635–48.

Roberts DL, Anstey AV, Barlow RJ *et al*. U.K. guidelines for the management of cutaneous melanoma. Br J Dermatol 2002; 146:7–17.

Scottish Intercollegiate Guidelines Network (SIGN). Cutaneous melanoma. A national clinical guideline. Edinburgh: Scottish Intercollegiate Guidelines Network (SIGN), 2003.

Thompson JF, Scolyer RA, Kefford RF. Cutaneous melanoma. Lancet 2005; 365(9460):687–701.

CHAPTER 11

Surgical management of skin cancer

Sajjad Rajpar, Jerry Marsden

OVERVIEW

- Clinicians treating skin cancer and pre-cancerous lesions must be well versed with the entire selection of diagnostic and therapeutic (both surgical and non-surgical) procedures so as to be able to tailor treatments to individual circumstances.
- The great majority of diagnostic and curative surgical procedures can be carried out under local anaesthetic in the ambulatory care setting.
- Surgical specimens must always be sent for histological investigation.
- Suspected melanomas should be excised in their entirety with an elliptical excision.
- A punch or incisional biopsy can be used to establish a diagnosis in lesions suspected to be non-melanoma skin cancer or pre-cancer.
- Excisional surgery remains the most common means of curing skin cancer surgically, although curettage and cautery can be a useful for pre-cancerous lesions, and small basal cell carcinoma (BCC) and squamous cell carcinoma by experienced operators.
- Mohs' micrographic surgery is the most precise method of excising skin cancer, and is particularly useful for ill-defined, and recurrent BCC.
- Complications after skin cancer surgery are uncommon, and include haemorrhage and infection.

Surgical procedures are carried out for both diagnosis and treatment of skin cancer (Table 11.1). The great majority can be performed under local anaesthetic in the ambulatory care setting. With suitable precautions, frail, elderly and anticoagulated patients can be treated safely. The choice of procedure depends on the site and type of lesion and the goal of the surgery. It is essential to form a clinical differential diagnosis before performing a diagnostic procedure, as histological results should always be interpreted in the clinical context. If the histological diagnosis is at odds with the clinical impression, then this must be resolved by discussion between clinician and pathologist. Negative biopsy results in the face of compelling clinical evidence of cancer or pre-cancer should be treated with caution, and further biopsies or complete excision of the lesion should be considered.

Table 11.1 Summary of surgical interventions for the diagnosis and treatment of skin cancer and pre-cancerous lesions

	AK or Bowen's disease	BCC	SCC	Melanoma
Diagnostic procedures				
Punch biopsy	✓	✓		
Incisional biopsy	✓	✓	✓	
Excisional biopsy	✓	✓	✓	✓
Curative procedures				
Curettage and cautery	✓	✓*	✓*	
Excision with narrow margins	✓			
Excision with wide margins		✓	✓	✓
Mohs' micrographic surgery		✓	✓	

*Avoid unless operator experienced and lesion small (< 1 cm) and low-risk – see text.

AK, Actinic keratosis; BCC, basal cell carcinoma; SCC, squamous cell carcinoma.

Diagnostic procedures

Punch biopsy

Punch biopsies are performed using a disposable device, the tip of which is a sharp circular cylinder (of varying diameters) that can bore up to 7 mm into the skin (Fig. 11.1). This releases a small cylinder of tissue that is separated and sent off for histological analysis. The resultant defect can be closed with a suture or packed and left to heal by secondary intention. Operators should be aware of important structures, such as nerves and blood vessels, beneath the biopsy site.

Incisional biopsy

An elliptical excision is performed from the centre of the lesion to normal perilesional skin, down to the level of the subcutaneous fat (Fig. 11.2). The defect is normally closed with monofilament skin sutures. Incisional biopsies are superior to punch biopsies for histological diagnosis, as they provide a larger, full-thickness sample of the lesion and perilesional skin.

Shave biopsy

The most superficial layers of a lesion are shaved off using a blade or razor. Haemostasis of the base is achieved with electrical or chemical

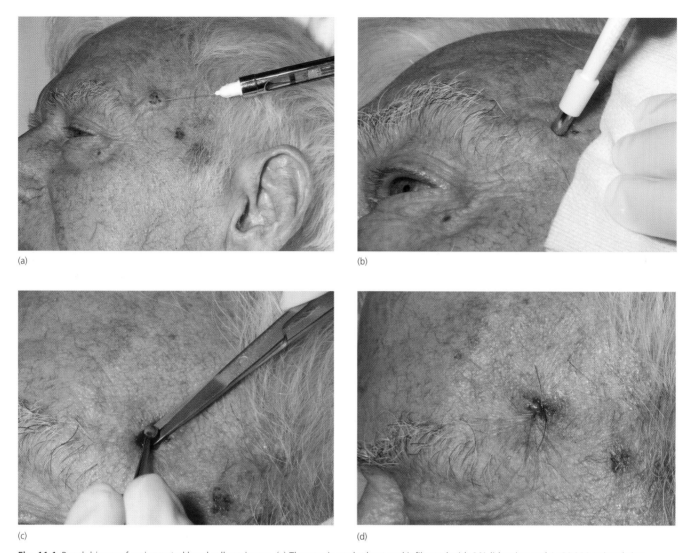

(a)

(b)

(c)

(d)

Fig. 11.1 Punch biopsy of a pigmented basal cell carcinoma. (a) The area is marked out and infiltrated with 2% lidocaine and 1:80 000 epinephrine. (b) The punch biopsy device is pressed down using a screwing motion. (c) A cylinder of skin is lifted with a skin hook or forceps and cut at the base with scissors. (d) The defect is sutured.

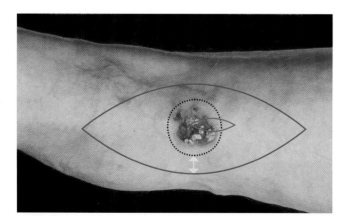

Fig. 11.2 An incisional biopsy (red) compared with a curative excision (blue) of a squamous cell carcinoma. A wide margin of normal looking skin is removed (yellow) along with the tumour to ensure areas of subclinical spread are excised. Note the clinical borders of the lesion (black).

cautery. Shave biopsies are appropriate for benign lesions that are protuberant above the skin surface, such as intradermal naevi. They are not suitable for diagnosis of lesions thought to be melanoma or other invasive skin cancer, since they may compromise subsequent histological measurement of tumour thickness.

Selecting the appropriate diagnostic procedure

Pigmented lesions

Suspected melanomas should be excised in their entirety with an elliptical excision taking 1–2-mm margins of normal perilesional skin. In certain exceptional situations, an incisional biopsy may have to be performed when the whole lesion cannot easily be removed because of size or location. An example would be a large lesion on the sole of the foot. Punch or shave biopsies should be avoided, as they may fail to diagnose melanoma because of sampling error. In the UK, suspected melanoma should not be excised or biopsied in primary care.

Non-melanoma skin cancer

Pre-cancerous lesions need to be biopsied if there is diagnostic doubt, failure to respond to treatment, or a possibility that invasive transformation to squamous cell carcinoma (SCC) has occurred. Diagnostic biopsies for basal cell carcinoma (BCC) and SCC are necessary if there is uncertainty about the diagnosis before definitive surgical treatment is offered, or if non-surgical treatments are being used. Negative biopsy results in the face of compelling clinical evidence of skin cancer should be treated with caution.

An incisional biopsy is preferred for ulcerated lesions and for SCC, as this enables a deeper sample that contains normal skin around the lesion to be obtained, aiding pathological analysis. Punch biopsies are acceptable for suspected pre-cancerous lesions and BCC. In the UK, most biopsies performed in primary care are likely to be on pre-cancerous lesions.

Curative procedures

The goal of treating skin cancer is to remove the tumour in its entirety together with any micro-metastases with acceptable cosmetic results and minimal functional morbidity. Conventional excisional surgery remains the most common means of treating skin cancer surgically, although curettage and cautery can be used in certain situations.

Surgical excision

Excisional surgery for skin cancer is generally performed by dermatologists and plastic surgeons who are part of a skin cancer multidisciplinary team. The benefits of excisional surgery over non-surgical treatments such as radiotherapy are that it can be completed in one visit, the whole lesion is available for histological analysis, and excision margins can be analysed to ensure the tumour is completely excised.

For both SCC and BCC, a margin of normal skin must be excised with the tumour, to ensure that any subclinical extension is adequately removed (Fig. 11.2). For BCC the deep margin is usually subcutaneous fat. For SCC the deep margin is usually periosteum, perichondrium, muscle or muscle fascia. The margins used are those that should result in complete excision of the primary lesion and vary with the type and size of skin cancer. Typical lateral margins are 6–10 mm for SCC and 4–8 mm for BCC. For melanoma, the entire lesion will usually have been excised in the primary diagnostic excision. Definitive treatment with wider excision is then necessary. The size of wider lateral excision margins varies from 1 to 3 cm, according to the Breslow thickness of the melanoma (Box 1.1; Figs 1.2 and 10.1). The deep margin is always muscle or muscle fascia. The surgical defect may be closed directly, with a skin flap or with a skin graft (Fig. 11.3). A skin flap is the use of adjacent skin to cover the defect, whereas a skin graft is the use of skin from a distant site.

Curettage and cautery

Curettes can be used to 'scoop out' a superficial and well-demarcated lesion in one piece, or 'scrape' through a lesion layer by layer (Fig. 11.4). Often, a combination of both techniques is applied, with the central

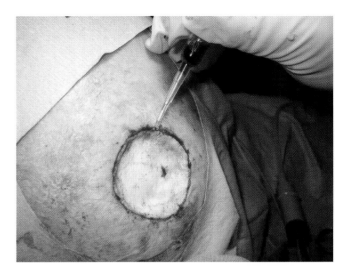

Fig. 11.3 A skin graft on the scalp being fixed with tissue glue.

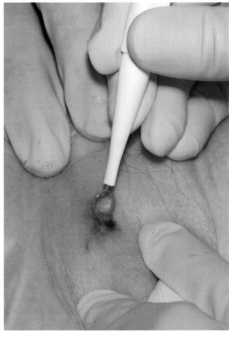

Fig. 11.4 Curettage of a small superficial basal cell carcinoma. Multiple cycles of curettage and cautery are required to ensure subclinical extensions are adequately treated.

bulkier area of a lesion scooped out, after which the periphery of the defect is scraped until all abnormal tissue is removed. Modern disposable curettes comprise an extremely sharp ring attached to an ergonomic hand piece. By virtue of their sharpness, these devices make it difficult to feel the difference between normal and abnormal tissue compared with traditional spoon-shaped curettes, which allowed for cleavage through a tissue plane. Curettage is performed under local anaesthetic, and haemostasis is achieved with chemical or electrical cautery. The time required for healing varies according to the depth of the wound that is created.

Curettage is most useful for benign superficial lesions such as viral warts and seborrhoeic keratoses. It can also be used to treat actinic keratosis (AK) and Bowen's disease, particularly for isolated lesions that are very hyperkeratotic or unresponsive to non-surgical treatments. The 5-year recurrence rates for Bowen's disease treated with curettage and cautery are between 10 and 20%. Small (< 10 mm) well-demarcated BCC and SCC can also be treated with curettage and cautery, and 5-year recurrence rates of 5 to 10% have been reported in selected populations treated by experienced operators. Success is highly operator dependent, and multiple cycles of curettage and cautery are required once the main tumour mass is debulked to ensure occult peripheral extensions are treated. A major limitation of curettage in the treatment of skin cancer is that the tissue obtained for histological analysis consists of fragments, which makes it impossible to exclude SCC when AK or Bowen's disease are curetted, or to be sure that margins are clear when BCC or SCC are treated. For these reasons, the authors favour excisional surgery over curettage for BCC and SCC.

Mohs' micrographic surgery

Mohs' micrographic surgery (MMS) (named after Frederick Mohs, the pioneer of this technique) is the most precise method of excising skin cancer and is used in specialist centres for the treatment of certain tumours, mostly BCC (Box 11.1). The lesion is excised, mapped and analysed immediately under the microscope. Further excision is undertaken in areas where residual tumour is seen. This is repeated until the field is tumour free. This ensures that all tumour-containing tissue is removed, whereas unaffected tissue is spared.

MMS is most useful for ill-defined or infiltrative BCC (Fig. 6.5), where occult strands that are not visible to the naked eye may extend well beyond the main tumour. This technique is also useful for lesions near critical structures such as the eyelids, where conservation of tissue is desirable. Because of its precision, MMS is associated with the best cure rates for BCC. However, availability of MMS is poor in the UK, as it is a highly skilled procedure that is very labour and time intensive.

Post-operative complications

Serious complications after surgery for skin cancer are uncommon (Table 11.2). Haemorrhage requiring intervention affects < 1% of cases, and usually develops in the first 24–48 h. Increased rates of haemorrhage have not been consistently demonstrated in anticoagulated patients provided the International Normalized Ratio is ≤ 3

Box 11.1 **Relative indications for Mohs' micrographic surgery**

BCC and SCC
- Ill-defined clinical outline
- Proximity to vital structures, e.g. the eye
- Infiltrative histology or perineural invasion
- Tumours recurring after surgery or radiotherapy

Rare tumours
- Dermatofibrosarcoma protuberans
- Desmoplastic melanoma; recurrent lentigo maligna
- Other tumours with subclinical contiguous local invasion

Table 11.2 Complications of surgery for skin cancer

Short-term complications	Long-term complications
Haemorrhage	Paraesthesia
Infection	Atrophic, widened or hypertrophic scars
Paraesthesia	Nerve palsy
Suture reaction	
Wound dehiscence	

Table 11.3 Incidence (%) of wound infection after cutaneous surgery varies by type procedure and by body site. (From Dixon AJ et al. Dermatol Surg 2006; 819–26)

Procedure	Incidence
Curettage	0.7
Simple excision	0.5
Skin flap	3.0
Skin graft	8.7

Location	Incidence
Face	0.8
Below knee	6.9
Groin	10.0

at the time of surgery; hence anticoagulation is not usually discontinued. Post-operative capillary bleeding may settle with firm pressure for 10 min. Arterial bleeding is unlikely to respond to this, and may lead to the formation of a painful haematoma. This requires the wound to be opened and for bleeding to be controlled.

Wound infection affects 1–2% of cases, but the exact rate varies with the type of procedure, whether the lesion is ulcerated, and body site (Table 11.3). Clinical features of wound infection are pain, erythema and purulent exudate. Late signs are necrosis, dehiscence and toxaemia. Increasing pain and tenderness 3–5 days after surgery suggest infection and should prompt inspection of the wound, microbiological investigation and antibiotic therapy. Cigarette smoking delays wound healing, and it is important to dissuade patients from smoking until sutures are removed. Numbness around the scar is common, and can last from a few weeks to several months. Scars may be lumpy and erythematous at first, partly as a reaction to dermal sutures, although most fade and flatten with time.

Further reading

Bolognia JL. I. Biopsy techniques for pigmented lesions. Dermatol Surg 2000; 26:89–90.

Lawrence C. An introduction to dermatological surgery, 2nd edn. Edinburgh: Churchill Livingstone, 2002.

Miller SJ. II. Biopsy techniques for suspected non-melanoma skin cancers. Dermatol Surg 2000; 26:91.

Robinson JK, Hanke WC, Sengelmann R et al., eds. Surgery of the skin. St Louis, MO: CV Mosby, 2005.

CHAPTER 12

Non-surgical treatment of skin cancer

Sajjad Rajpar, Jerry Marsden

OVERVIEW

- Clinicians treating skin cancer and pre-cancerous lesions must be well versed with the entire selection of diagnostic and therapeutic (both surgical and non-surgical) procedures so as to be able to tailor treatments to individual circumstances.

- It is essential to be certain of the diagnosis before embarking on any non-surgical treatment for non-melanoma skin cancer and pre-cancerous lesions.

- Radiotherapy is a useful alternative to surgery for basal cell carcinoma (BCC) and squamous cell carcinoma.

- Actinic keratoses (AKs), Bowen's disease and superficial BCC respond to several non-surgical treatments. Cryotherapy is the cheapest option, but only practical if there are fewer than five lesions. 5-Fluorouracil, imiquimod and photodynamic therapy are more practical if there are multiple lesions or if a large area of field change needs to be treated. Topical diclofenac is suitable only for treating AKs.

Pre-cancerous lesions are by definition limited to the epidermis, and this makes them amenable to a variety of non-surgical interventions (Table 12.1). Similarly, some of these treatments are effective for superficial basal cell carcinoma (BCC). However, radiotherapy is the only reliable alternative to surgery for invasive lesions such as squamous cell carcinoma (SCC) and nodular and infiltrative BCC. As a rule, it is essential to be confident of the diagnosis before embarking

Table 12.1 Summary of non-surgical interventions for the treatment of non-melanoma skin cancer and pre-cancerous lesions

	AK or Bowen's disease	BCC	SCC
Cryotherapy	✓	✓	
Radiotherapy	✓	✓	✓
5-FU cream	✓	✓*	
Diclofenac gel	✓†		
Imiquimod cream	✓‡	✓*	
Photodynamic therapy	✓	✓*	
Laser resurfacing	✓		

*Superficial BCC only.
†AK only.
‡Not licensed for AK or Bowen's disease in the UK at the time of writing.
AK, Actinic keratosis; BCC, basal cell carcinoma; SCC, squamous cell carcinoma; 5-FU, 5-fluorouracil.

upon any non-surgical treatment, as treatment may preclude the opportunity to obtain an accurate histological diagnosis at a later stage. A biopsy should therefore be considered if there is diagnostic difficulty or a possibility that malignant transformation has taken place in pre-cancerous lesions.

Topical treatments

Topical treatments can be applied by patients or carers at home and are suitable for the treatment of actinic keratosis (AK), Bowen's disease and superficial BCC when alternative treatments are less favourable, e.g. when there are multiple lesions to treat, when there are lesions below the knee where healing is poor, and when a single large area of affected skin is treated, often referred to as an area of field change. Certain key principles should be observed when prescribing topical treatments (Box 12.1).

Diclofenac

Topical diclofenac is available in the UK as a 3% gel in hyaluronic acid. Twice-daily application for 60–90 days reduces the number of AKs by 50–70%. The exact mechanism of action is uncertain. Although it is well tolerated and local reactions are mild, durability of benefit is unclear and, as for other topical treatments, there are no data to show that it reduces subsequent risk of SCC. Topical diclofenac formulations licensed for musculoskeletal pain lack hyaluronic acid are not effective for AK.

5-Fluorouracil

5-Fluorouracil (5-FU) is available as a 5% cream in the UK and is useful for the treatment of AK, with reported response rates of 70–90%, and for Bowen's disease, with reported response rates as high as 90%. It can also be used for the treatment of small superficial BCCs (Table 12.2). 5-FU inhibits thymidylate synthase leading to arrest in DNA synthesis and cellular necrosis. For best results in treating AKs it should be applied to the whole area being treated, e.g. the forehead, since subclinical lesions will respond. At the licensed dose of twice a day for 4 weeks, an inflammatory reaction typically arises at the end of the first week and is occasionally quite vigorous (Fig. 4.5). Patients should be forewarned and advised to continue treatment even if lesions become red or crusty, cut down the frequency of application if soreness is excessive, and stop if an open sore develops.

Box 12.1 **Key principles of using topical treatments for non-melanoma skin cancer and pre-cancerous lesions**

- Suitable for superficial lesions (thin AK, Bowen's disease and superficial BCC) if alternative treatments are less appropriate, e.g. multiple lesions, lesions below the knee, field change
- Hyperkeratotic (scaly or heavily keratinizing) lesions are unlikely to respond and are better treated surgically
- It is essential to be certain of the diagnosis before treatment. This requires a biopsy for Bowen's disease and superficial BCC, and for AK if lesions are not clinically typical
- Lesions located on the scalp and face respond best. Avoid for lesions that are very close (< 1 cm) to the eyes
- Clear instructions should be provided both verbally and in writing
- Treatment should be applied to the lesion and to 0.5–1 cm of perilesional skin
- If a large surface area needs treatment with 5-FU or imiquimod (e.g. whole scalp), then one segment should be treated at a time to prevent an overwhelming inflammatory reaction
- The presence of an inflammatory response increases the likelihood of efficacy for 5-FU and imiquimod
- It is necessary to monitor response to treatment at regular intervals
- Treatment should be stopped if a weeping, painful erosion develops
- SCC or BCC must be excluded (by biopsy) if lesions do not respond to one full course of treatment, or recur rapidly after apparent clearing
- Patients should be followed up 12 weeks after treatment to ensure that the lesion has responded, and at 12 and 24 months to assess for recurrence

AK, Actinic keratosis; BCC, basal cell carcinoma; 5-FU, 5-fluorouracil; SCC, squamous cell carcinoma.

It is useful to restrict application to one site at a time, and move to another area once the skin has healed, which usually takes another 4 weeks. 5-FU cream is sometimes used on alternate days for 8 weeks or twice a week for 12 weeks, in an attempt to cut down the severity of local reactions, although efficacy may be compromised. The addition of a topical steroid to minimize local reactions has been suggested, although its effectiveness or effect on clearance rates have never been established. Treatment with topical 5-FU is most effec-

tive for AKs on the head and neck, and longer treatment may be required for lesions at other sites.

Imiquimod

Imiquimod is a novel drug from the imidazoquinolone group that activates host immunity against tumour cells, leading to an anti-tumour cytotoxic T-cell response. In the UK and Australia, 5% imiquimod cream is licensed for superficial BCC at a dose of five times a week for 6 weeks. It is also licensed for AK in the USA, at a dose of twice a week for 16 weeks. Clearance rates for superficial BCC appear to be around 80%, although up to 20% of lesions may recur at 3 years. Recurrence rate beyond 3 years is not known. Although data from a randomized controlled trial comparing imiquimod with surgery for superficial BCC are awaited, imiquimod appears to be less effective than surgical excision for superficial BCC.

As with 5-FU cream, erythema, flaking, scabbing, pruritus and soreness at the site of application are common (Fig. 12.1). The extent of these side-effects is greater with increased frequency of applica-

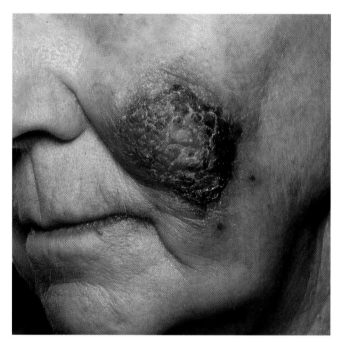

Fig. 12.1 Treatment with imiquimod may produce a pronounced inflammatory reaction.

Table 12.2 Advantages and disadvantages of 5-fluorouracil and imiquimod for superficial BCC

Advantages	Disadvantages
Avoidance of a major surgical procedure	Requires pretreatment biopsy to confirm diagnosis
Avoidance of surgical scar	Treatment may be prolonged – 6 weeks (imiquimod) to 10 weeks (5-FU)
Treatment can be carried out at home	Cure rates may be lower than with surgical excision
Reasonable to good cosmetic outcome	Lack of histological confirmation of clearance
Can treat multiple lesions	May require post-treatment biopsy to confirm adequacy of response
	Risk of severe inflammatory reactions and systemic upset
	Risk of chronic ulceration and slow wound healing
	Cost effectiveness uncertain

tion. Brisker side effects are associated with a better response, and it needs to be made clear to patients that an inflammatory response is, to a certain extent, desirable. Titrating therapy to the inflammatory response is often required; if side-effects are excessive, then the frequency of application needs to be reduced or temporarily stopped. Several subclinical lesions may become inflamed and noticed for the first time when a photodamaged field is treated. Rarely, inflammatory dermatoses such as psoriasis may be exacerbated by imiquimod, and systemic release of cytokines can lead to flu-like symptoms. Cosmetic results are good, although residual erythema and postinflammatory dyspigmentation can occur.

Radiotherapy

Radiotherapy is effective in curing BCC and SCC (Table 12.3). Radiotherapy is also used in the adjuvant setting for tumours that are at high risk of recurring after surgery, and for incompletely excised tumours. Superficial X-rays or electrons are used depending on the location and depth of the tumour. The total radiation dose is divided into several fractions that are delivered over a number of days. A typical regime for a BCC may involve treatment on 5 days a week for 1 or 2 weeks. Radiotherapy is used mainly for lesions on the head and neck, as treatment on other areas (particularly the legs) is associated with slower healing, poorer cosmetic results and increased rates of radiation necrosis (Fig. 12.2).

Radiotherapy is an option for patients > 65 years old. Younger patients are likely to have sufficiently long life expectancy for radiation-induced skin cancer to be a concern. Indications for radiotherapy include very large tumours or tumours situated on the eyelid, canthi, nose, ears and lips, as surgery may lead to unacceptable cosmetic or functional morbidity. Radiotherapy may also be considered in patients who are unfit for an operation or have a strong preference to avoid surgery.

Treatment is relatively painless, and each fraction takes 10–20 min to deliver. Immediate side-effects include erythema and soreness, which usually settle after 4–6 weeks and can be ameliorated with a mild topical steroid. Lesions may ulcerate, crust and scab before healing. Most patients rate the short-term cosmetic result of radiotherapy as good or excellent. In the long term, irradiated skin usually becomes pale and atrophic. Patchy hyperpigmentation and telangiectasias may also develop after several years (Fig. 12.3).

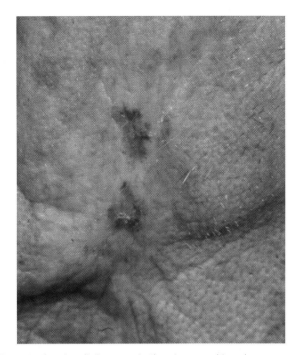

Fig. 12.2 Chronic radiation necrosis. There is an atrophic and hyperpigmented scar with areas of skin breaking down that may be confused with recurrent basal cell carcinoma (BCC). This has developed several years after radiotherapy for BCC.

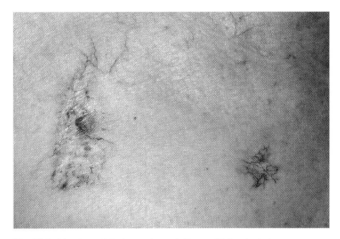

Fig. 12.3 Atrophy, patchy hyperpigmentation and telangiectasias may develop several years after radiotherapy for skin cancer.

Cryotherapy

The open spray technique with liquid nitrogen is commonly used to treat AKs (Fig. 4.4), Bowen's disease and superficial BCC. Lesions can be treated quickly, usually within one or two treatments. However, several complications are recognized that are dependent on the site treated and the duration of freeze, and should be balanced against the potential benefits (Table 12.4). Patients must be consulted properly, and provided with written aftercare information.

Between 70 and 80% of AKs can be cured with cryotherapy, though hyperkeratotic lesions respond poorly, as keratin acts as an insulator. A single freeze of about 5 s is often adequate for thin AKs

Table 12.3 Advantages and disadvantages of radiotherapy

Advantages	Disadvantages
Suitable for lesions around the eye, nose, ears and lips	Multiple visits required
Suitable for large lesions	Histological assessment cannot be made
Suitable for deep lesions	Not suitable for lesions on the trunk and limbs
Painless	Long-term risk of skin atrophy, dyspigmentation, telangiectasias and radionecrosis
Good cosmetic results	Only suitable for patients >65 years old as there is a small risk of radiation-induced skin cancer Shortage of radiotherapy units in the UK

Table 12.4 Advantages and disadvantages of cryotherapy

Advantages	Disadvantages
Quick	Acute side-effects (in the first 48 h) include pain, oedema, blister formation
Cheap	Delayed side-effects (days to weeks) include secondary infection, delayed wound healing and chronic ulcer formation (particularly on legs)
Multiple lesions can be treated in one visit	Long-term side-effects (years) include hypopigmentation, scarring, alopecia
No anaesthetic required	Less effective for heavily keratinized lesions
Suitable for elderly and infirm	Cure rates operator dependent as inexperienced operators tend to undertreat
Healing usually rapid on the head and neck	

with minimal hyperkeratosis. With these parameters, side-effects are minimal and cosmetic outcomes are acceptable. Thicker AKs may require freeze durations of 5–10 s, although this increases the incidence of blistering and hypopigmentation (Fig. 12.4).

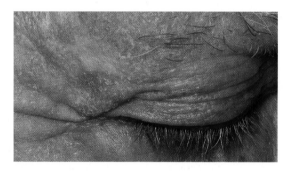

Fig. 12.4 Hypopigmentation is a complication of cryotherapy, seen here after treatment for actinic keratosis. The incidence of hypopigmentation increases with increasing freeze times.

Longer freezes, typically between 10 and 15 s, are required for Bowen's disease, as the full thickness of the epidermis is affected, and for superficial BCC, where the superficial dermis is also involved. At these freeze durations, oedema, weeping and blistering are common. Healing can take up to 3–4 months on the legs of elderly ladies, where Bowen's disease is common. Cryotherapy should be used judiciously in this situation – topical chemotherapy, curettage and photodynamic therapy (PDT) may be better options.

Photodynamic therapy

5-Aminolaevulinate cream or methyl-aminolaevulinate cream are applied to lesions under occlusion for 4 h. These are preferentially taken up by dysplastic cells, where they saturate the haem biosynthesis pathway leading to an excess of intracellular protoporphyrin IX (PpIX), an endogenous photosensitizer. Light, at a wavelength capable of activating PpIX (usually in the red spectrum), is then applied for 10–60 min (depending on the power of the light source). Photoactivated PpIX produces highly reactive free radicals and singlet oxygen intermediates that lead to cell death. Cure rates for AK, Bowen's disease and superficial BCC are in the order of 70–95%. PDT is particularly useful for wide areas of actinic damage such as the scalp, for large lesions and for lesions located on the lower legs. Cosmetic results are superior to cryotherapy. PDT is labour intensive, and currently only available in specialist dermatology units.

Further reading

Dawber R, Colver G, Jackson A. Cutaneous cryosurgery – principles and clinical practice, 2nd edn. London: Martin Dunitz, 1997.

Gupta AK, Davey V, Mcphail H. Evaluation of the effectiveness of imiquimod and 5-fluorouracil for the treatment of actinic keratosis: critical review and meta-analysis of efficacy studies. J Cutan Med Surg 2005; 9:209–14.

Szeimies RM, Morton CA, Sidoroff A, Braathen LR. Photodynamic therapy for non-melanoma skin cancer. Acta Derm Venereol 2005; 85:483–90.

CHAPTER 13

Skin cancer – an Australian perspective

Lachlan Warren, Karyn Fuller

OVERVIEW

- Australia has the highest incidence of skin cancer in the world.
- The incidence of melanoma and non-melanoma skin cancer continues to increase in Australia.
- Rates are higher in lower latitudes, in residents born in Australia and those with poor tanning ability.
- The majority of skin cancers are treated by surgical excision and are managed in the primary care setting.
- The SunSmart programme is conducted by the Cancer Council Australia as a primary prevention strategy to curb the rising incidence of skin cancer.
- Problems with delivery of skin cancer treatment in Australia include fragmentation of care and coordination, advertising and entrepreneurial activities to induce attendance for procedures, and inequality of service provider delivery and accessibility.

Australia has the highest incidence of skin cancer in the world, where it outnumbers other forms of cancer by more than 3 to 1. Non-melanoma skin cancer (NMSC) is the most diagnosed and most expensive cancer in Australia, costing more than AU$232.2 million per year. Over 1% of Australians are treated for a NMSC during any 12-month period.

Epidemiology

Melanoma

Australia has the highest global incidence and mortality rates of melanoma. In 2001, incidence rates were 46 per 100 000, four times that of the UK, and mortality rates were 5.5 per 100 000, double that of the UK. In Australia, melanoma is the most common cancer among those aged 15–44 years and the second most common cause of cancer death in that age group. Each year, 850 people die of melanoma and there is an annual loss of > 10 000 person-years of life before 75 years of age. The incidence rate for melanoma among males and females increased between 1991 and 2001 on average by 2.1% and 1.2% per year, respectively. Mortality rates increased by 0.5% and 0.2% per annum for males and females, respectively, between 1996 and 2001.

Non-melanoma skin cancer

In 2002–2003 there were an estimated 374 000 NMSC cases in Australia, compared with an estimated 60 000–100 000 in the UK. This

is greater than five times the incidence of all other cancers combined and is increasing (Table 13.1). The male to female incidence ratio is 1.9 to 1 for squamous cell carcinoma (SCC) and 1.4 to 1 for basal cell carcinoma (BCC). In Australia 200 people die each year from skin cancers other than melanoma.

Risk factors

It is widely accepted that exposure to ultraviolet (UV) radiation is a major factor in the development of skin cancer. Residents born in Australia have at least twice the risk of skin cancer compared with British migrants, suggesting that a major determinant of lifetime risk for skin cancer is sun exposure during childhood and adolescence. Among Australian-born people, the rates of skin cancer are highest in those with fair skin and a poor tanning ability. Skin cancer in Aboriginal and Torres Strait Islander Australians is rare.

A comparison of the yearly variation of UV index for four locations of different latitudes [Chilton (UK), Melbourne (South Australia), Brisbane (Central Australia) and Darwin (North Aus-

Table 13.1 Age-standardized rates per 100 000 (95% confidence intervals) by tumour type for surveys, 1985, 1990, 1995 and 2002

	1985	1990	1995	2002	% increase 1985–2002
BCC					
Males	735 (623, 847)	849 (767, 931)	955 (879, 1034)	1041 (936, 1158)	42
Females	593 (491, 694)	605 (537, 674)	629 (568, 696)	745 (662, 839)	26
Persons	657 (585, 729)	726 (673, 780)	788 (739, 840)	884 (816, 957)	35
SCC					
Males	209 (149, 268)	338 (287, 389)	419 (372, 473)	499 (430, 580)	139
Females	122 (75, 169)	164 (139, 199)	228 (193, 268)	291 (242, 349)	139
Persons	166 (128, 204)	250 (220, 281)	321 (292, 354)	387 (344, 434)	133

From *The 2002 National Non-Melanoma Skin Cancer Survey*. A report by the NCCI Non-melanoma Skin Cancer Working Group. Melbourne: National Cancer Control Initiative, 2003. Copyright Commonwealth of Australia, reproduced with permission.

tralia)] shows that there is a significant increase in UV exposure with increasing proximity to the equator (Fig. 13.1). It follows that inhabitants of Northern Australia, being closer to the equator (< 29°S), have a much higher incidence of skin cancers, between three- and fourfold, than those in Southern Australia (> 37°S) (Table 13.2).

Management

In contrast to the UK, the majority of skin cancers in Australia are treated in the primary care setting. More advanced and complex disease is managed by secondary care specialists. Skin cancers are the most common cancers managed by Australian general practitioners, with > 800 000 patient encounters per year.

Melanoma

Survival after the diagnosis of melanoma in Australia is high, with 89% survival at 5 years and 86% at both 10 and 15 years. These rates reflect both improved early diagnosis and a trend with time to thin-

Table 13.2 Age-standardized rates per 100 000 for basal cell carcinoma (BCC) and squamous cell carcinoma (SCC) in Australia by latitude in 2002 (95% confidence intervals)

Latitude	BCC Rates	SCC Rates
Low (North Australia)	1662 (1439–1921)	794 (639–985)
Medium (Central Australia)	959 (859–1071)	432 (368–506)
High (South Australia)	547 (454–659)	232 (177–306)

Skin cancer rates are increased in areas that are closer to the equator. (From *The 2002 National Non-Melanoma Skin Cancer Survey*. A report by the NCCI Non-melanoma Skin Cancer Working Group. Melbourne: National Cancer Control Initiative, 2003. Copyright Commonwealth of Australia, reproduced with permission.)

ner melanoma. The median Breslow thickness of melanoma at diagnosis in Australia is now 0.75 mm.

Non-melanoma skin cancer

In Australia about 256 000 people were treated for BCC and 118 000 for SCC during 2002. Seventy-three per cent of BCCs and 79% of SCCs were treated by surgical excision (Table 13.3), which is the treatment of choice as it produces the highest cure rates. Radiotherapy, curettage with cautery and cryotherapy, respectively, deliver increasingly lower cure rates. Mohs' surgery is indicated for skin cancers that are located on the central face and periorificial areas, recurrent disease, incompletely excised NMSC, high-risk histological types and large or ill-defined tumours. Between 2005 and 2006, 5012 Mohs' procedures were conducted in Australia. Curative radiotherapy is usually reserved for a small minority of NMSC for which surgery would be inappropriate.

Cryotherapy achieves high cure rates for actinic keratoses. It is also used for lower risk primary tumours on the trunk and limbs, including Bowen's disease, primary superficial or small papular BCC,

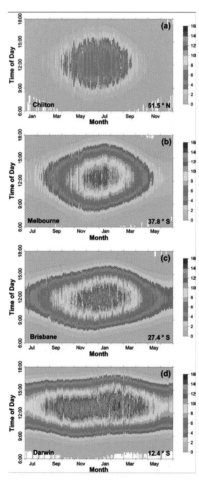

Fig. 13.1 Three-dimensional colour plots of the yearly variation of ultraviolet (UV) index for four locations of different latitudes: Chilton (52.8N) (a), Melbourne (37.88S) (b), Brisbane (27.58S) (c) and Darwin (12.48S) (d). There is a significant increase in UV exposure with increasing proximity to the equator. (From Gies. Photochemistry and Photobiology 2004; 79:32–9. Copyright Commonwealth of Australia, reproduced with permission.)

Table 13.3 Treatment by histological type of skin cancer in 2002

| Treatment type | Histological type | | | | | |
	BCC	%	SCC	%	Total	%
Surgical excision	695	72.8	325	78.7	1020	74.6
Cryotherapy	105	11.0	30	7.3	135	9.8
Curettage or diathermy	84	8.8	35	8.5	119	8.7
Other management*	20	2.1	3	0.7	23	1.7
Treatment not stated	51	5.3	20	4.8	71	5.2
Total	955		413		1368	

From *The 2002 National Non-Melanoma Skin Cancer Survey*. (A report by the NCCI Non-melanoma Skin Cancer Working Group. Melbourne: National Cancer Control Initiative, 2003. Copyright Commonwealth of Australia, reproduced with permission.)
*Includes radiotherapy (=6), imiquimod (=4), fluorouracil (=3), no treatment given (=10). No lesions were treated with photodynamic therapy, interferon or laser therapy.

keratoacanthomas and small primary well-differentiated SCC, although this is different from UK practice. 5-Fluorouracil cream is commonly prescribed for widespread actinic keratoses. Curettage and cautery is used in small, primary superficial BCC on the trunk and limbs, small SCC where surgical excision is impractical, and for keratoacanthoma and Bowen's disease. Imiquimod cream and photodynamic therapy are a treatment option for nodular and superficial BCC, although exact roles await the results of further studies and long-term cure rate assessment.

Who treats skin cancer in Australia?

Skin cancers are treated by a variety of different medical practitioners in Australia, including general practitioners, dermatologists, plastic surgeons, general surgeons and radiotherapists (Table 13.4). Each group has different levels of training, experience and therapeutic approaches. General practitioners utilize surgery and occasionally cryotherapy and curettage, whereas dermatologists use most modalities of treatment. The pivotal position occupied by general practitioners in the Australian health system accounts for the fact that they diagnose and manage most suspicious skin lesions in Australia, particularly in rural areas.

A new development in Australia is the skin cancer clinic (Fig. 13.2). Skin cancer clinics are commonly managed by large 'corporate' chains or smaller independent operators. They are serviced by general practitioners or non-specialist doctors from a variety of backgrounds. Universal health insurance ('Medicare') provides financial rebate for consultations and procedures, supporting these clinics. There are increasing numbers of skin cancer clinics in Australia, and there is controversy about the type and quality of their services. Mainstream general practice, funded overwhelmingly by fee-for-service rather than capitation, is threatened by fragmentation.

Table 13.4 Number and percentage of basal cell carcinoma (BCC) and squamous cell carcinoma (SCC) lesions by clinic type in 2002

Clinic type	BCC	%	SCC	%
GP	355	37.2	211	51.1
Skin cancer clinic	119	12.5	33	8.0
Dermatologist	272	28.5	84	20.3
Plastic surgeon	113	11.8	38	9.2
Other surgeon	35	3.7	17	4.1
Hospital	12	1.2	2	0.5
Other	21	2.2	16	3.9
Not stated	28	2.9	12	2.9
Total lesions	955		413	

From *The 2002 National Non-Melanoma Skin Cancer Survey*. (A report by the NCCI Non-melanoma Skin Cancer Working Group. Melbourne: National Cancer Control Initiative, 2003. Copyright Commonwealth of Australia, reproduced with permission.)

Plastic surgery and dermatology are threatened by encroachment into their domains of practice. However, there are insufficient dermatologists to cope with demand and the geographical distribution of dermatologists and plastic surgeons precludes them managing most patients.

In Australia there are no barriers to working in skin cancer medicine in primary care. There are limited training opportunities for generalist doctors and there is no accreditation or defined standards. The Skin Cancer Society of Australia was formed in 2005 to address these problems. Their aim, in consultation with specialist groups, is to develop training, standards, accreditation, audit and research to ensure that skin cancer medicine in primary care provides optimal health outcomes for patients.

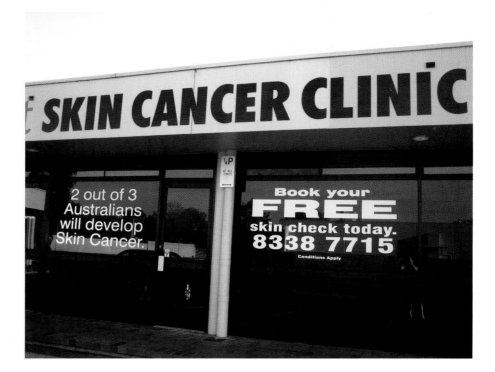

Fig. 13.2 Skin Cancer Clinic. There is controversy about the type and quality of service provided by skin cancer clinics, which are commonly managed by large 'corporate' chains or smaller independent operators.

Prevention

Prevention and early detection of skin cancers are critical control measures. If Australians reduced their exposure to UV radiation it has been estimated that the incidence of skin cancer could be potentially reduced by >90%. There is some evidence that programmes raising public awareness and earlier diagnosis have resulted in greater numbers of thin tumours diagnosed, with improved survival rates for melanoma.

The Australian National Health Care Policy acknowledges that the prevention of skin cancer is a societal responsibility. There are Australian standards governing UV radiation protection incorporated into numerous legislative bills. These include standards for a variety of sun protective products (sunscreens, photoprotective apparel, sunglasses) and occupational standards for sun exposure. The Cancer Council ran a health promotion programme named 'Slip! Slop! Slap!' from 1980 to 1988 and continue with their SunSmart programme (Fig. 13.3). Recommendations include wearing protective clothing, using a sunscreen with appropriate sun protection factor, wearing a hat and avoiding the sun. Studies have reported higher knowledge levels about skin cancer and higher levels of sun protection in Australia compared with other countries. The SunSmart programme includes a National SunSmart Schools programme, which is a policy based accreditation programme. Their Sporting and Recreational Organisation Sponsorship Project is funded by the State government

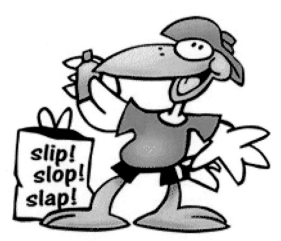

Fig. 13.3 Slip! Slop! Slap! Campaign logo.

tobacco taxes to promote the SunSmart message in these sectors. They also target outdoor workers including farmers and fishermen in their Sun Protection and Outdoor Workers Project encompassing policy guidelines and on-site education sessions. SunSmart encourages local governments to ensure shade provision is included in Council policies regarding facilities and events. A Mass Media Project with a National Skin Cancer Action week at the commencement of summer serves to maintain skin cancer as a health issue on the public agenda.

Vitamin D

UV radiation is responsible for cutaneous synthesis of vitamin D3, critical for calcium homeostasis and skeletal maintenance. Benefits for other types of cancer, bone disease, autoimmune diseases, hypertension and cardiovascular disease have been reported. Outcome results from these studies are based on dietary supplementation of vitamin D. The main source of vitamin D for Australians is exposure to sunlight. Levels of serum vitamin D3 vary according to the season and are lower at the end of winter. In Australia 23% of women have a marginal vitamin D deficiency and 80% of dark-skinned veiled women have a definite deficiency. Further work is necessary to define an adequate vitamin D status, and avoid widespread vitamin D deficiency due to excessive photoprotection for skin cancer prevention.

Further reading

Clinical Practice Guidelines. Non-melanoma Skin Cancer. Guidelines for Treatment and Management in Australia. National Health and Medical Research Council. October 2002. Available at http://www.nhmrc.gov.au/publications/_files/cp87.pdf

Clinical Practice Guidelines. The Management of Cutaneous Melanoma. National Health and Medical Research Council. December 1999. Available at http://www.nhmrc.gov.au/publications/_files/cp68.pdf

National Cancer Control Initiative. The 2002 National Non-Melanoma Skin Cancer Survey. A report by the NCCI Non-melanoma Skin Cancer Working Group. Melbourne: National Cancer Control Initiative, 2003.

Nowson C, Margerison C. Vitamin D intake and vitamin D status of Australians. Med J Aust 2002; 177:149–52.

Staples MP, Elwood M, Burton RC et al. Non-melanoma skin cancer in Australia: the 2002 national survey and trends since 1985. Med J Aust 2006; 184:6–10.

SunSmart Evaluation Report. Anti-Cancer Foundation of South Australia. October 2001. Available at http://www.cancersa.org.au/cms_resources/documents/Resources/SunSmart/SunSmartEvaluationReportIntro.pdf

CHAPTER 14

Cutaneous metastases and rare skin cancers

Sajjad Rajpar, Jerry Marsden

OVERVIEW

- The most common solid organ malignancies to metastasize to the skin are those of the lung, colon, breast, ovary and kidney.
- Merkel cell carcinoma is a rare primary skin cancer that is believed to be caused by excessive exposure to ultraviolet light. It is the third leading cause of death from skin cancer.
- Mycosis fungoides is the most common type of cutaneous T-cell lymphoma. It generally runs an indolent course in most patients and is often mistaken for benign inflammatory dermatoses such as eczema, tinea and psoriasis.
- Angiosarcoma and Kaposi's sarcoma are malignancies of endothelial cells. The latter most commonly occurs in the context of HIV infection, and is caused by human herpesvirus 8.
- Cutaneous Paget's disease of the nipple is unilateral, and mimics nipple eczema. There is a strong association with underlying ductal carcinoma of the breast. Extramammary Paget's disease is found in the anogenital area or axillary skin, and is associated with malignancies of the bowel, reproductive and urinary system.

Cutaneous metastases and a selection of rare primary skin cancers are discussed in this chapter. Despite its large surface area and rich blood supply, the skin is a relatively infrequent site of metastasis from primary solid organ or haematological malignancies. However, due to the sheer number of non-cutaneous primary cancers, skin metastases are regularly seen in clinical practice. Melanoma, squamous cell carcinoma (SCC) and basal cell carcinoma account for 99% of primary skin cancers. Several rare skin cancers collectively account for the remainder. Some are highly aggressive, but may appear misleadingly benign, such as cutaneous angiosarcoma, which may initially be mistaken for a simple bruise. Others, such as mycosis fungoides, may also be mistaken for benign disorders, but are reasonably indolent in their behaviour.

Cutaneous metastases

Solid organ and haematological malignancies may metastasize to the skin, usually through lymphatic and haematogenous routes. Metastases to the skin are significantly less common than metastases to visceral organs such as the lungs and liver, and are present in only 1–5% of patients with metastatic malignancies. After melanoma, in order of frequency, the most common primary cancers to metastasize to the skin are lung, colon, breast, ovary and kidney. Occasionally the presence of cutaneous metastases may be the first sign of the underlying cancer.

Dermal metastases present as painless, skin-coloured to erythematous papules and nodules (Fig. 14.1). Subcutaneous metastases are mobile lumps which may initially be mistaken for cysts, although a history of a new and growing lesion should suggest a malignant diagnosis. Lesions are often multiple, and a skin biopsy confirms the diagnosis as the histological features resemble those of the primary tumour. Thorough history taking, general physical examination, analysis of tumour markers and imaging studies may also help identify the primary tumour.

Management of cutaneous metastases is centred around treatment of the underlying cancer. Specific lesions that have become symptomatic can be treated with laser or electrosurgery, excision or local radiotherapy. The presence of cutaneous metastases nearly always denotes a poor prognosis, but nonetheless does not necessarily indicate rapid progression of disease.

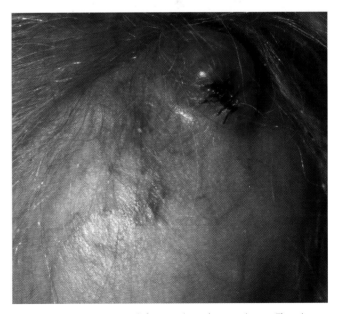

Fig. 14.1 Cutaneous metastasis from a primary lung carcinoma. There is a well-demarcated erythematous nodule on the scalp. A biopsy has been performed.

Merkel cell carcinoma

Merkel cell carcinoma (MCC) is rare, although because of its high mortality it is the third leading cause of death from skin cancer after melanoma and SCC. MCCs occur on sun-exposed sites of older individuals, suggesting excessive ultraviolet exposure is pathogenic. Lesions appear as rapidly growing, indurated hemispherical purple to red papules or nodules that may ulcerate (Fig. 14.2). The clinical features are non-specific, and the differential diagnosis includes SCC, lymphoma (usually B cell), nodular melanoma or cutaneous metastasis. Histologically, MCC resembles small cell lung cancer and immunostaining helps differentiate the two. Treatment involves wider surgical excision and adjuvant radiotherapy. Despite aggressive local treatment, lymph node metastases develop in 55% of patients and solid organ metastases in 34%. The overall 5-year survival rate is 50–60%. MCC is an area of intense interest, and a new staging system and clinical trials are in development.

Cutaneous lymphomas

The skin has important immune functions and contains resident and trafficking immune cells. Malignancies may develop from any type of skin immune cell, although the most frequent are extranodal non-Hodgkin's lymphomas arising from cutaneous T or B lymphocytes.

Cutaneous T-cell lymphoma

The cutaneous T-cell lymphomas (CTCL) are a heterogeneous group of more than 10 disorders that together account for 5% of non-Hodgkin's lymphomas. The most frequent CTCL is mycosis fungoides (MF), which has an annual incidence of 0.5 per 100 000 population. The prevalence is much higher due to its in-

dolent course and relatively good prognosis. MF most commonly presents in the sixth decade and is slightly more common in males and Blacks.

Four stages of disease progression are recognized: patches, plaques, tumours then nodal/visceral involvement. All may eventually co-exist, but patches are usually the earliest form, and are flat or just palpable scaly erythematous lesions which may be circular or annular. Plaques are thicker and more palpable than patches (Fig. 14.3). Lesions may be pruritic and, unlike most inflammatory dermatoses, are fixed in position. Patches and plaques of MF are nonetheless frequently misdiagnosed as eczema, tinea or psoriasis, and patients may be treated for these disorders for several years before the correct diagnosis of MF is reached. The definitive diagnosis is made on skin biopsy, although multiple biopsies are frequently required. MF is not curable, so the aim of treatment is safe and effective control of symptoms. For patches and plaques of MF, this includes emollients, topical steroids and phototherapy. The most important practical point is that treatment is palliative, and is driven by clinical need, not histopathological diagnosis. This is fundamentally different from non-cutaneous lymphomas. For example, MF may transform, often locally, to much higher-grade anaplastic large T-cell lymphoma, a diagnosis that would normally suggest chemotherapy. However, a low-key palliative approach will normally provide safe and effective disease control.

Progression of patches and plaques of MF is slow and sometimes absent, hence the 5-year survival rate is in the range of 85–95%. Patients with early patch or plaque stage MF, i.e. < 10% of body surface involvement, have a long-term survival indistinguishable from a normal population. Extensive ulcerated painful tumours with lymphadenopathy may result, and infiltration of the entire skin can lead to erythrodermic MF or Sezary syndrome. MF cells will then be found in the blood. Survival for most is limited to 1–3 years, with significant disease-related immunosuppression. Treatment involves palliative chemotherapy, radiotherapy and experimental treatments such as mini-allografts and immunotherapy.

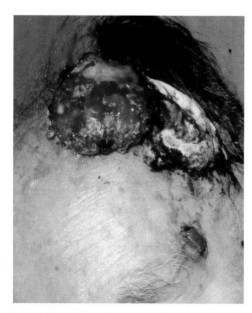

Fig. 14.2 Merkel cell carcinoma. There is a rapidly growing fungating nodule on the scalp, with extensive local spread. Merkel cell carcinomas tend to be aggressive and have high mortality rates.

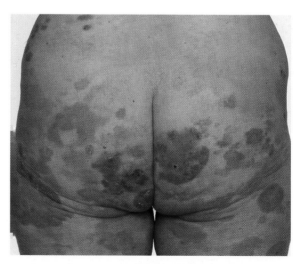

Fig. 14.3 Mycosis fungoides (MF). There are scaly patches and plaques, which are discoid and annular. Patches and plaques of MF are often mistaken for inflammatory disorders such as psoriasis, tinea and eczema.

Cutaneous B-cell lymphoma

Cutaneous B-cell lymphomas (CBCL) are less common than CTCL. Follicle centre lymphomas present as grouped erythematous nodules on the trunk or head and neck. Lesions are responsive to radiotherapy, and 5-year survival rates are generally >90%. Anaplastic large B-cell lymphomas affect the legs of elderly individuals, particularly females (Fig. 14.4). These lesions present as red dermal nodules and tend to disseminate early on, leading to a poor outlook.

Cutaneous sarcomas

Sarcomas are malignancies that arise from connective and soft tissues. Most sarcomas arise in the bone and muscle, although a small number arise from skin structures.

Angiosarcoma

Angiosarcomas are malignancies of endothelial cells that line blood and lymphatic vessels. They are very rare tumours, with an estimated annual incidence of 0.5 per million population. The most common location is the scalp and upper face, appearing as a red to purple macule (Fig. 14.5). They can easily be mistaken for a bruise, but the lesion is fixed, often >5–10 cm, normally without a satisfactory history to explain it. Angiosarcomas can also occur post radiotherapy, and in long-standing lymphoedema either in the lower legs or after mastectomy. Angiosarcomas are very aggressive and the 5-year survival rate is in the order of 10–40%. Treatment includes wide excision and adjuvant radiotherapy.

Kaposi's sarcoma

Kaposi's sarcoma is a type of angiosarcoma that is caused by human herpesvirus 8. In the UK, the majority of cases occur in patients with defects of T-cell-mediated immunity, either iatrogenic (from immu-

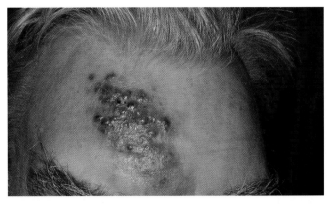

Fig. 14.5 Angiosarcoma. These highly aggressive tumours are rare and most frequently occur on the head and neck of elderly White males. They may initially be mistaken for a bruise, but tend to progress rapidly.

nosuppressive medications) or secondary to HIV infection. Kaposi's sarcoma presents as red, purple or black macules, papules and nodules (Fig. 14.6). The gastrointestinal and respiratory tract may also be affected. Anti-retroviral treatment often brings about significant improvement in HIV-associated Kaposi's sarcoma, although systemic chemotherapy is occasionally required. Treatment is palliative.

Dermatofibrosarcoma protruberans

These tumours are believed to arise from fibroblasts or histiocytes, and have an annual incidence in the order of 1–3 per million population. Most lesions occur on the trunk or head in young to middle-aged adults. Lesions appear as slowly growing, irregular rubbery dermal subcutaneous lumps, often present for several years. Initially, they may look like large dermatofibromas, but the lumps begin to spread and coalesce to produce more extensive skin infiltration. They are often thought to be scars, or misdiagnosed as 'cysts', and can reach 5–10 cm in diameter before the correct diagnosis is reached. Excision using Mohs' micrographic surgery provides a very high chance of cure. Metastasis is rare, and usually associated with transformation of long-standing disease to fibrosarcoma.

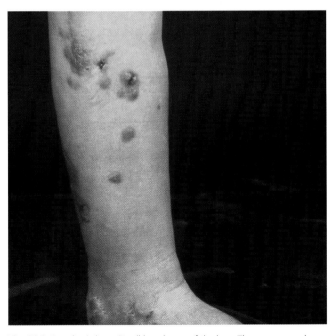

Fig. 14.4 Anaplastic large B-cell lymphoma of the legs. There are several erythematous nodules on the legs.

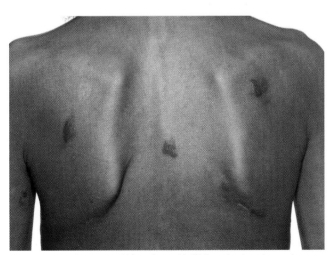

Fig. 14.6 Kaposi's sarcoma. This patient with HIV has developed several red-brown macules, plaques and nodules on the skin and the oral mucous membranes. Kaposi's sarcoma is caused by infection with human herpesvirus 8.

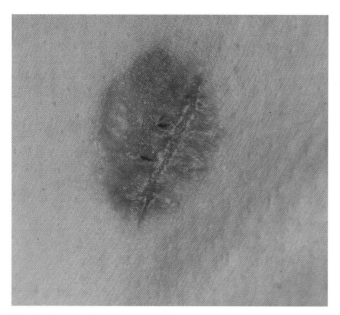

Fig. 14.7 Dermatofibrosarcoma protruberans. There is a slow-growing firm, indurated plaque on the trunk, with a scar running through the lesion from an incisional biopsy. Early lesions are often mistaken for a scar.

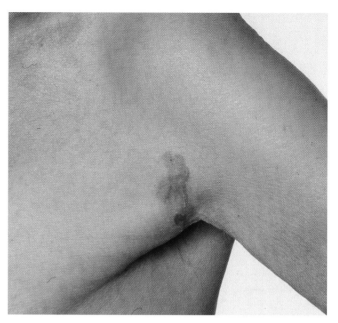

Fig 14.8. Extramammary Paget's disease. There is a well demarcated erythematous plaque that is eroded inferiorly.

Adnexal tumours

Benign and malignant tumours may arise from hair follicle structures and apocrine, eccrine and sebaceous glands. These lesions are collectively known as adnexal (or appendageal) tumours. More than 20 varieties are recognized, most of which present as slow-growing, 5–10-mm dermal nodules (Fig. 7.4).

Cutaneous Paget's disease

Paget's disease of the nipple presents as a unilateral scaly erythematous plaque around the nipple that may be mistaken for eczema. The vast majority (>90%) of women with Paget's disease of the nipple will have an underlying invasive or *in situ* ductal carcinoma of the breast. Therefore, patients with suspected Paget's disease of the nipple should be referred to a breast surgeon for triple assessment that includes physical examination, mammography and nipple biopsy.

Extramammary Paget's disease (Fig. 14.8) occurs in the axillary or anogenital area, and is histologically identical to Paget's disease of the nipple. Lesions present as well-demarcated erythematous plaques which may be scaly, macerated or eroded. Lesions are often mistaken for irritant dermatitis or candidal intertrigo. Twenty-five per cent of

lesions are associated with an underlying cancer of the urothelium (kidney, ureter and bladder) or lower gastrointestinal tract or genital tract (uterus, ovary, prostate). Other primary sites should also be considered, especially breast cancer in those with axillary disease. Occasionally, the underlying cancer may be in contiguity with the disease on the skin. The remaining lesions are presumed to be primary cutaneous adenocarcinomas. Management involves a search for an underlying malignancy and surgical excision of the Paget's disease. It is very prone to recur, and again Mohs' micrographic surgery is likely to provide higher rates of cure than conventional wide excision. Radiotherapy alone is less effective than surgery.

Further reading

Lookingbill DP, Spangler N, Helm KF. Cutaneous metastases in patients with metastatic carcinoma: a retrospective study of 4020 patients. J Am Acad Dermatol 1993; 29:228–36.

Mendenhall WM, Mendenhall CM, Werning JW et al. Cutaneous angiosarcoma. Am J Clin Oncol 2006; 29:524–8.

Swann MH, Yoon J. Merkel cell carcinoma. Semin Oncol 2007; 34:51–56.

Whittaker SJ, Marsden JR, Spittle M et al. Joint British Association of Dermatologists and U.K. Cutaneous Lymphoma Group guidelines for the management of primary cutaneous T-cell lymphomas. Br J Dermatol 2003; 149:1095–107.

Index